THE *Write*
PRESCRIPTION

THE *Write*
PRESCRIPTION

Telling Your Story to Live With and Beyond Illness
Judith Hannan

To my mother and father

Contents

Stories are antibodies against illness and pain.

—Anatole Broyard

The body is a Bodhi tree

The mind a standing mirror bright

At all times polish it diligently

And let no dust alight.

—Yuquan Shenxiu

Foreword

by Charles Barber

In this age of evidence-based medicine, there is an incontrovertibly proven treatment that in the prevailing environment of "units of care" and "episode-of-care payment reimbursement rates" is unfortunately little paid attention to—namely, the simple truth that writing and telling stories about illness is good for your health. The psychologist James Pennebaker at the University of Texas has spent a career conducting a series of clinical trials that prove *that writing heals*—in an astonishing number of ways, among them, lowering blood pressure, lifting moods, improving the immune system, and facilitating recovery from traumatic events. The sum total of the evidence is that telling stories about illness is, or should be, a healthcare treatment unto itself.

It is odd then that there are few books or manuals to help patients tell their experience of illness. But then again, this is perhaps not so surprising—the current medical system largely thrives on the silence of patients, or what is euphemistically called "compliance." Into this void arrives Judith Hannan's *The Write Prescription*, which lays out a series of practical and wise steps to break the silence of those who have suffered. It is less a writing book than a "let's get writing" book. It takes the process stepwise, from micro to macro. "Part One" presents a series of writing prompts that facilitate close observation, point of view, dialogue, and free association. "Part Two" helps the patient transform those finite observations and material into scenes, involving journeys, families, conversations, conflicts. "Part Three" encourages the writer to write about the medical experience and the medical system itself—doctors and nurses, insurance, technology. Throughout, Judith Hannan occupies the role of the encouraging expert, informed by her various roles as patient, family member, and writer of illness stories.

Although eminently clear-eyed and pragmatic in its tone, *The Write Prescription* is, at its core, a radical book. The late doctor and writer Walker Percy wrote that scientific experts are the true "princes of the age." In the modern technological era we have, bit by bit, relentlessly and willingly ceded ever more parts of ourselves to the appointed experts. "*They* know about science, *they* know about medicine, *they* know about everything in the cosmos, even me," Percy wrote.

Judith Hannan, with this book, is entreating you, the reader, to become no less than an expert in yourself. This is unheard of in the managed care environment. Doctors and the medical system are important and essential of course, but when it comes to the *experience* of illness and treatment, only the patient knows the exact and relevant truth. Here Judith Hannan is asking you to dig down hard and find, and then tell, and then maybe even publish, your story. This has been found to be a particularly worthy form of noncompliance.

Introduction

I was pregnant with twins, going for my first visit to the OB/GYN. After giving her my medical history, I caught a glimpse of my new chart. At the top, I saw a Venus symbol, ♀, and alongside this skeletal goddess was a downward pointing arrow with an adjacent notation: ♀↓bc 55. A woman, my mother; dead from breast cancer at age fifty-five.

That's not my mother, I wanted to say. Even though eight months later this highly skilled doctor would prevent me from becoming a downward-pointing arrow as well, she would have been a far less able narrator of my life. What if she had written: *Judith's mother died of breast cancer at the age of fifty-five.* And what if, after writing that, the doctor would have been prompted to write that fifty-five is so young. Then maybe she would have asked me how it felt to be a mother without having a mother and learned about all the growing up I had had to do since my mother died. But after I said my few words, it was time to move on to the next question and my mother's story and mine stayed inside, adding to the weight of my pregnant belly.

I can see how the full story of my mother's life could have been considered irrelevant from a medical perspective. I was seeing this particular doctor because I was a thirty-eight-year-old woman expecting twins, officially high risk, and she was the best in her field. Eight months from that first visit, I would never see her again. It's not as if I showed any curiosity about her life beyond her qualifications. I knew she was Latina, that she got her training when the "M" in medical school could just as easily have stood for male. If she placed a reassuring hand on my arm now and again, that was enough, although I don't remember if she did or not. More important to me was the determination I saw on her face trying to save my life when I began to hemorrhage during delivery. Neither of us was thinking about each other's stories at that moment.

Still, that chart. It's been twenty-two years since I saw that Venus symbol and I still feel it like a slap. Where is my mother's flesh, her core? What did *my* symbol look like?

The art of gathering and telling patients' stories is about putting a body onto those skeletal symbols, adding a heart, and injecting a soul. Narrative Medicine is the official term used in academia and medical schools. Taking a history is about receiving a story. But narrating illness is not just for doctors; it's for anyone who has been a patient, a caregiver, a spouse, or a child. People who were writers before illness entered their lives instinctively turned to the page, to, as Emily Rapp explains so beautifully in her book, *The Still Point of the Turning World*, note in the midst of grief "...the ways in which writing about the experience from the inside creates something new, namely a safe or safe-ish place to rest. A net, a landing point, a dock from which to view the turbulent and troubled water without having to wade in it every moment of every day." Creating narrative is the opposite of disease.

Without words, illness isolates us. As the late author Reynolds Price wrote in *A Whole New Life*, his chronicle of his treatment for a spinal cord tumor, "I needed to read some story that paralleled, at whatever distance, my unfolding bafflement—some honest report from a similar war..." So stories are both antibodies for ourselves and for others. I know how Price felt. In 2001, after my then-eight-year-old daughter Nadia finished her successful treatment for Ewing's sarcoma, one of our first nonmedical outings was to our neighborhood bookstore in search of books in which we could find ourselves—she, a young patient; me, a mother of an ill child. We were searching a desert which held no thirst-quenching elixir for her and very little for me. Books about death and grief were more plentiful; perhaps the extreme tragedy makes it more impossible to resist telling the story. I read these stories because I had looked into that dark abyss, but I was released.

Survival tells a different tale. I was not looking for an ode but a messy and uncertain narrative. I knew I had to write my own story. At the time, I was still so connected to illness and hospitals that my writing was self-centered, the style overblown because, while the storm that had roiled my emotional ocean had passed, the waves shuddering through me were still large and white-capped. It was not much more than a disguised daily journal, not very different from my obstetrician's

Venus symbol and downward pointing arrow because I wasn't telling a story about people but about IVs, scans, chemo drugs, scars, etc.

I saved those initial ramblings—their rawness would be necessary to the final narrative—until I was ready to weave them into a larger picture. I waited three years. I was ready, I thought, to meet myself on the page, to write the pain with honesty and without flinching. But the person I met there wasn't very nice. I wasn't being brutally honest, just brutal. I was writing without compassion and so without any hope of discovering just how I had been transformed.

It would be another five years before I could sit down to tell the story that needed to be told. It turned out to be different from the one I had assumed I wanted to read eight years earlier. Indeed, if I had read that one, it would have been more damaging than helpful. It would have kept me tethered to the past as if it were still the present. The essential component to any good narrative is surprising yourself with a discovered truth. Without moments when you say "aha" you are venting, not healing. My moments came when I stopped making myself the center of all my thoughts, when I found compassion for the people I was used to blaming or being angry with.

I wrote my first book, *Motherhood Exaggerated,* as a route to personal transformation and as a mirror for others. But there is another reason. For the past several years, I have volunteered at the Children's Museum of Manhattan helping homeless mothers write about personal experience. Some of their most profound work lets the reader into their lives during moments when no one can see them. It could be when a special interaction with a child confirms for them that they are good mothers, or when they have conquered a negative impulse or experienced a time of despair. It could paint a portrait of what happens in the middle of the night when darkness and the soul have a private conversation. "Look at me; I am here," they say.

As an author, I have come to realize I am not only a storyteller but a story-receiver. Stories are brought to me at book readings or in classes like presents that, for so long, could find no one to open their wrappings and lift out the precious treasures. First the giver says thank you. Then he or she speaks.

"My son had cancer. He didn't make it. Now I'm writing. My other son has psychological problems. You understand."

"My son has a serious mental disorder. My stepdaughter had cancer and her mother wasn't very much help."

"My husband's esophagus ruptured."

"I have an incurable leukemia. I've only told three people, not even my children. Your book is such a gift to me."

"I'm going to make my husband read this book. I've never had an ill child, but I am a mother and my husband has no idea what that means."

Readers tell me about their daily hurdles, the major traumas—the moment that will grab us all someday when the path we thought we were walking alters course, like the stairs at Hogwarts that keep changing the place of their landing.

The purpose of this book is to help those dealing with illness to birth more stories—whether to share with others or just as a gift for themselves. There is no dearth of excellent books about writing. Why is it necessary to add one that deals specifically with writing about illness? Isn't it really just an extension of personal narrative? In fact, the roots for *Motherhood Exaggerated* were set down in Nancy Aronie's Chilmark Writing Workshop which is about writing from all chambers of the heart. But those roots needed more places to go. They needed to be trained to grow through illness, a territory not known for its nourishment. The language of illness, medicine, healing, death, grief, and survival is still being written and we should all have the chance to contribute to it.

I don't believe we can move on from trauma, but we need to be able to move *with* what has happened to us. Writing can be a companion that takes our arm as we walk. It can heal or nourish or fortify. A recently completed study showed that walking through an area of trees and greenery allows your brain to recover from fatigue. Here, you are invited to walk within your own story, following your mind as it journeys through what has happened, marveling at the scenery of your revelations and your insights.

How To Use This Book

Writing about a moment in life filled with trauma and uncertainty can be daunting. What has happened is so big and so life-altering, we can become defeated before we start. The prompts in this book are intended to be gateways which take you into small moments and single events. Some are not even specifically about illness. By approaching your story in small bites, your appetite to keep writing will grow. Which direction you choose to go in once you have entered your story is up to you. The only goals are the ones that you set; you may be writing just for yourself, as a way to share with family, and/or because you want the larger world to read your story. None of the prompts will insist that you use a specific form, correct punctuation, or have a certain word count. When writing samples are provided they are only for guidance, not to copy or to dictate the right way to respond to the prompt.

Whenever I work from a book of prompts, I flip around, sometimes opening to a page at random, sometimes reading several suggestions before finding one that speaks to me that day. While there is a loose order to the prompts (one that I changed often during the writing process), you are encouraged to create your own order.

The book is divided into three sections. The first includes a series of warm-ups that would benefit both the new and more practiced writer. They will not only help you get started but expand your way of thinking, particularly when your subject refuses to fit easily into your container of words. Keep these strategies in mind as you explore the prompts in the second section, which ask you to relate specific scenes and events. The final section gives you the opportunity to write about the medical system—what you liked and what you didn't. You will find, though, that there is significant overlap between these sections. The most important strategy to keep in mind is to not limit or stop yourself once you have passed through the gateway.

Many of these exercises can be done multiple times and from different stages in your life. Each chapter usually has a number of prompts for you to select from. After choosing one you can either choose another or move onto a different chapter knowing you can always return at a later date. Follow your own instincts. By wringing each prompt for varying stories and perspectives, you will find that your narrative of illness will be woven into the larger setting of your life experiences, relationships, and even physical atmosphere.

Similarly, what you choose to do with your writing is up to you. Perhaps just writing is enough. If you want to create a more polished piece that others will read, there is a section at the end on revision and submission.

Your writing is an excellent way to share your experiences with family members and friends, either as a way to communicate what you never articulated before or to offer lessons. It can provide an avenue for talking about heretofore hidden or unresolved sentiments. Be careful, though. If the material is potentially hurtful or confusing, do not just hand it to your intended reader and walk away. Be prepared to stay and talk and explain.

The wider public is also hungry for stories of the experience of illness. Maybe you are considering creating a piece for publication. I encourage you to share your stories but also add a note of caution here. Be very selective about who you first share your work with. A critical comment, suggested rewrites, or a dismissive remark don't only hurt, they can keep you from facing the page again. Choose someone loving and supportive and, until you have the confidence, someone not in your story.

There are also many support groups with websites that encourage people to share their stories online. Spending a day researching some of these options would be a good idea if you want both to relate your own experiences and to read the narratives of others in similar circumstances.

Part I

Getting Started

By deciding to tell your story, you have chosen to embark on a voyage that I hope will be exciting; but it will not always be comfortable or familiar. When my father was first diagnosed with Alzheimer's disease, he began losing control over his speech. Words, he said, would run away just as he was about to grab them. Writing can be like that. You know your story, but the minute you pick up a pen or pencil or place your hands on your keyboard, the words are gone—snatched away by fear, resistance, self-doubt. Often, we are overwhelmed by all that we have to say. We tackle the mountain before finding our footing on the path of the gentle lower slope.

The following chapters will help get you started. They are both warm-ups and suggestions on how to face your subject when approaching it head-on is too formidable. Perhaps, before you start writing about your experience with illness, you need to develop your confidence as a writer with exercises and subjects no less personal but not as daunting. If you are ready to dive right in, these exercises can take you as deep as you wish to go, or you may just wish to skim this first section or use it as a reference as you proceed through later chapters. And when the inevitable happens and you run into a wall, you can always return to these chapters to prime your pump again. Remember, proceed at the pace that feels right to you.

Just Show Up

When my kids were little, I learned to write anywhere. While I sat on the floor with a toddler playing dress up, a baby in my lap and her twin in a bouncy seat, I could eke out a few sentences, maybe a paragraph. If I put the kids near water and sand I could buy a little more time. I always carried a notebook with me and wrote in school lobbies and doctors' offices, at horse shows and gymnastic meets. These days, I have a number of spaces within my empty nest where I think I can find the best words; not surprisingly, I still find myself drifting back to the couch in the playroom; or else I go to the local library when cleaning the bathtub seems like a more appealing option than writing.

The point is, there is no perfect condition for writing except that you make yourself present. A few key decisions must be made, however. If you prefer to write by hand, you have to choose between a pen or a pencil, lined or unlined paper, loose or bound. If a computer, do you prefer a PC or Mac, a simple word processor program or one of the many creative writing software packages. Do you need access to an outlet or are you diligent about keeping your computer charged?

Do you prefer solitude or company or both, depending upon your mood?

That's it for the necessities. But if you have a dedicated space to write, dress it up and make it comfortable. Pin inspiring quotes or pictures onto a bulletin board. If music helps you write, build a playlist. Wherever you are, be prepared. Always keep a small notebook with you, so if you find yourself waiting forty-five minutes for a family member's plane to land, you can write in the airport lounge. Don't wait for the perfect time and place; make the time and place perfect.

It would be ideal to write every day, but for many of us, that expectation can backfire. Set realistic goals, particularly if you have never made writing a priority before. If all you can make time for are fifteen to twenty minute sessions a few days a week, then that's how you begin.

Your Assignment

Go shopping for pens, pencils, paper, etc. Set up a file on your computer. Get a small notepad you can carry with you or make sure you have a note-keeping app on your cellphone for when inspiration strikes in the waiting room or on the bus to work.

Getting Here

You've arrived at your desk, library, coffee shop, couch. What are you thinking? Are you excited, or not sure what you've gotten yourself into? Right at this moment your mind is engaged in a running narrative. Usually, we try not to pay attention to our inner monologues. Too often they are filled with doubts and self-criticism, or else we are criticizing others. We are beset by memories that float up uninvited, or our list of chores waves itself before our eyes, blocking our view of what is in front of us. Our brains just can't help themselves; they scream for attention.

But there are times when we should listen. Like right now. Pay attention to your thoughts and feelings, the stream of consciousness narrative that comes from your belly rather than your brain. At the very first writing workshop I ever took, the prompt was "Getting Here." My internal monologue went something like this:

> *Getting here. Getting here? What does she mean by that? I drove. I don't think that's what we're supposed to write about. It's not very interesting. I should have walked. It's only a mile. But I'm never ready on time. I drove the yellow Jeep Wrangler with no top or windows. A mud-spattered, sand-filled Martha's Vineyard car. Does that put me in*

the same category as these aging hippies? I hated being a hippie. I liked having long black hair, dressing in ethnic-looking clothes, playing the guitar, and singing "Hey Mr. Tambourine Man." But I hated all that love stuff. I wasn't feeling it. Like in those consciousness-raising groups where we're supposed to be so honest and open up to each other. People were mean, and if you weren't like them they said you were aloof and stuck-up. Oh God. Is this workshop going to be like that? Who cares how I got here. Why did I come? People kept telling me I should write. Based on what? The grant proposals I wrote, or those direct mail pieces that stuffed up people's mailboxes? I don't think I will be writing about the benefits of arts education here. I must have had a reason for coming. Because I love stationery stores and the sound of pencil on paper. Because I've passed the sign to the Chilmark Writing Workshop for years. Because in third grade I was passed out of penmanship into the creative writing program. Because my mother had me write her thank you cards. Because I am a mother now and need to learn how to tell stories the way they were never told to me. Because I need some way to pry myself open.

Writing Prompt

- Now it's your turn. How did you get to this point? Why are you here, staring at a blank page or a blinking cursor? What were you thinking when you decided to buy this book, in the time between when you bought it and now? What are you thinking right now? What excites you or makes you fearful? Let all thoughts in, even the extraneous ones, like remembering you forgot to buy orange juice this morning. It's as important to know what thoughts are distracting you as those that are keeping you focused. Write for ten minutes without stopping. If you get stuck, repeat a previous sentence and see where it takes you the second time or keep writing "What am I thinking?" as many times as you have to before another sentence comes to you.

Free Association

One of my favorite children's books is *If You Give a Mouse a Cookie*. It is a one-thing-leads-to-another story that was great fun to read aloud to my kids. After asking for a cookie, a mouse asks his host for a glass of milk, then a straw, then a mirror to check for a milk moustache, and then scissors to trim his hair, and then on and on. I love the energy of the free association and arriving at unexpected situations, like asking for soap to wash a floor or a pen to sign a painting.

We free associate all the time—when we meet a stranger, look at an object, taste a food, hear a song, or enter a new circumstance. Usually, these associations happen so fast that we don't notice them and the process is abbreviated by our lack of attention.

Shortly after Nadia finished treatment, I had to serve jury duty. During a break, while we were waiting in the jury room, I became fixated on a coat stand in the corner. It was warm out, so there weren't any coats hanging from the metal hooks. I found it disconcerting, so I took out my notebook and wrote, "The coat stand reminds me of…" Here is what followed:

The coat stand reminds me of an IV pole, which reminds me of the kids riding on their poles down the hospital hallways, which reminds me of Nadia and her friend Akivah trying to sell their homemade hair growth tonic, which reminds me of the Passover seder we had in the hospital with a Hasidic family, which reminds me of my first-generation but very secular father knowing to bring his hat with him so he could cover his head, which reminds me that it wasn't my family who taught me about being a Jew, which reminds me of leading a "rock" service at our temple, which reminds me how much I loved singing into the mic, which reminds me that I haven't played my flute in a long time, which reminds me of my music stand which is as barren as the coat rack.

Writing Prompt

- Pick an object, a remembered moment, or a place, and begin to free associate by writing: The _____ reminds me of _____, which reminds me of... Don't overthink your selection, and begin writing immediately so you don't have time to anticipate where you will arrive. Again, don't stop writing. All associations are valuable. Write for a minimum of ten minutes but keep going for longer if you are still running strong.

Making Metaphor

Until I turned fifty, I had migraines every month. I was nauseated, my head pulsed, and my left eye felt swollen like it would pop from its socket. To get relief, I gentled my head down onto my pillow and spent hours concentrating only on emptying my pain into the bedclothes. I have a friend who suffers from migraines, and when she tells me one is coming on I should know right away what she is feeling, but her pain seems unreal to me. While I can describe what I felt for so many years, it is only a memory, an avatar of the real thing. Once pain or any sensation is gone, a selective amnesia occurs, perhaps for our own sanity. But there is another reason why I can't connect to my friend's pain. It's because there are no external clues to the dilation of blood vessels that has just begun in her head. None of my five senses have been put on alert. Conveying physical sensations, feelings, and emotions requires a different language, particularly in writing, when the narrator is not standing before you to offer even the tiniest physical clue.

This is where metaphor becomes a powerful tool for expressing the unseen and untouchable. A metaphor is simply a way of describing one thing by naming it as something else to which you make an association. For example, anyone walking into a hospital might see the same set of sliding glass doors, the reception desk, the warnings about hand washing; but in his essay, "The Lake of Suffering," from *Portrait Inside My Head*, Phillip Lopate wants us to see what he sees when he takes his daughter to the hospital, so he uses metaphor. "The hospital was like a space ship: no gravity, no up or down, white, weightless." In his book of essays, *Intoxicated by My Illness*, Anatole Broyard writes, "I imagined [my illness] as a love affair with a demented woman who demanded things I had never done before." The reader now knows that Broyard's writing will have edges, and some of them might scrape.

In *The Still Point Of The Turning World*, Emily Rapp writes about losing her son to Tay-Sachs Disease. Her great challenge is to describe the specificity of a feeling that threatens to be steamrolled by tragedy. She succeeds by turning to metaphor. The wail in her voice can be heard as real sound when she writes, upon receiving the diagnosis, "I had the sensation of skin falling away from bone."

Writing Prompt

- Create metaphors for whatever you have difficulty naming. To get you started, I have provided a list of open-ended phrases for you to complete. Continue making up more of your own.

> **EXAMPLE**: *The feel of a hospital gown on my skin is...fluttering moth wings.*

> *Watching you leave is...*

> *The dog barking all night is...*

> *A needle entering the skin is...*

> *The sound of the nurse's shoes...*

> *The waiting room...*

> *Fresh air on my face...*

> *The ringing of the telephone...*

> *The sound of his/her cry...*

> *The view from the window...*

- Use metaphor to describe aspects of your nature and emotions. You can also place yourself in contrast to another person. Clip images from magazines and make metaphor from what you see.

  > **EXAMPLE**: *I am the moon, suspended between the outstretched limbs of two trees.*

  > *I am the empty canoe on the still lake; you are the one who propels me and roils the water.*

- Write an extended metaphor for one feeling or emotion. Begin each line by naming what you are trying to describe, i.e., pain is…, bravery is …, patience is…, loneliness is…, loss is…, waiting is…, etc., and create a different metaphor for the same feeling for each line.

The Five Senses

A picture is worth a thousand words. It's such an oft-repeated adage that one could think that everything there is to know about a moment in time can be discerned through the eyes. But pictures are unreliable narrators. The truth of a photograph cannot be told just by looking at it, because each viewer imbues it with his or her own ideas, memories, perspectives. The same can be said about setting a scene in a story you are telling. If you only describe what the eye sees, you are limiting your understanding of the moment and the experience of the reader. In memoir particularly, you want that reader to feel what you feel and to know what you know, and that can happen only if you make use of all of your senses.

For example, you can describe a five-foot-eleven-inch man in a gray suit, blue-and-white striped shirt, tasseled loafers, a plain gold wedding band, curly salt-and-pepper hair, and a trim beard. But until you describe the quality of his handshake, the timbre of his voice, the movement of his eyes, the slight scent of antiseptic soap that wafts around him, he is not much more than a fairly well-dressed mannequin. If his hand is moist and his grip limp, if his voice is swallowed and directed at your left shoulder, if the bottle of Purell on his desk is the economy size, then he becomes a character who does not inspire confidence or intimacy.

Writing Prompt

• This is an exercise you can do as many times as you choose with as many scenes as you want and from any point in your life. The objective is to include all appropriate senses in what you are describing.

Once you have picked your scene, make a list of what you saw. Repeat the process but include only what you heard. For example, if you described seeing a woman walking across a wooden floor in high heels, you should be sure to include the speed and clack of those heels. Now, move on to smell, then touch, then taste. Even if a sense doesn't seem applicable, think hard to make sure you haven't let a detail escape unnoticed. Once you have your separate descriptions, blend them together to provide a full-bodied illustration of your scene.

Here is a brief example describing a walk I took in Central Park with my dogs on an early July evening:

WHAT I SAW

> *Fireflies at late dusk skimming the grass, in the brush, up in the trees*
>
> *Joggers, bike riders, dog walkers*
>
> *Paved pathways, gravel horse trails,*
>
> *My dogs*
>
> *A bat*
>
> *Cars, trucks, and buses coming through the east/west transverse and going down Fifth Avenue*
>
> *The sky on its way to midnight blue, my hand a silhouette against it*

WHAT I HEARD

> *Rubber soles of my shoes sticky on the damp pathway, crunchy on the gravel*
>
> *Rhythmic tread and heavy breathing of joggers coming up behind me, moving away*

Dogs barking, tags jingling

My dogs snuffling in the leaves, panting

Robins, finches, and sparrows singing their final song for the night

Horns, engines of traffic, radios playing rap, salsa, and talk radio through open windows

Rise of the wind playing more loudly in the leaves

Fireflies are silent

WHAT I FELT

Plastic handles of leashes, the grip making my left hand ache

Heat, at first welcome after the air conditioning of my apartment, now cloying

Coolness at the back of my neck when I lift up my hair

Surprise of raindrops, at first confused with the sweat prickling my arms

Wind across my increasing dampness, hair standing up from the chill

WHAT I SMELLED

Dead fish

THE SCENE

The fireflies drew me to Central Park. I have been drawn to these tiny beacons ever since they beckoned me years earlier, when Nadia was in remission, to walk among them without her by my side. These silent, flickering insects are not what I associate with New York City. Like hundreds of tiny Tinkerbells, they seem too delicate to survive the onslaught of noise from the cars, trucks, and buses exiting the park's transverse, the radios blasting a cacophony of rap, salsa, and talk radio. The smell is all wrong, too—not of green grass and chlorophyll but of dead fish and dumpsters. Joggers thud past focused on their inhales and exhales; bike riders ring their bells and curse at absentminded dog walkers trying to cross in front of them. My dogs pant in the heat which, at first, felt welcome after the air conditioning of my apartment, but is now suffocating. I lift my hair and the air cools the back of my neck. The light on Fifth Avenue must be red now because it becomes quiet enough to hear the robins, finches and sparrows singing their last song of the evening. A bat swoops low. The dogs snuffle in the leaves. I remain still, watching the fireflies, like burning snowflakes, skim the grass, float in and out of the brush, climb high into the oaks and maples. The sky is a deepening blue; my hand, when I lift it to brush away a mosquito, is in silhouette. The wind rises in a whoosh of sound like the exhale of an invisible being. It causes the tree limbs to dance as if they yearned to be set free from their roots. My arms prickle. I think it is from sweat. The air is so heavy with moisture it is impossible to mark the moment when it starts to rain. Then the first few drops of a squall begin to hit the ground, sending up puffs of dust. The wind against the increasing dampness of my skin and clothes makes the hair on my arms stand up from the chill. The traffic light changes, the rumble of tires and engines begins again, the friction of rubber against water like radio static. How is it that the fireflies appear so untroubled in their silent drifting? They are the ones in a true heightened state—flashing electricity, looking for sex. The noise, the wind, the rain, the dead fish smell—it is all outside of their universe and too much in mine. I grip the leash handles the way I used to grip Nadia's hand and run home.

Look Closely

Jennifer Roberts, a professor of the history of art and architecture at Harvard University, has a requirement that her students write a research paper on a single work of art. Before picking up a pen or pencil or turning on a computer, students must spend three consecutive hours studying their painting, to engage in what Roberts calls "deceleration, patience, and immersive attention," ("The Power of Patience," *Harvard Magazine*, Nov-Dec 2013). What the students gain from such observation is a recognition of patterns, relationships, coloration, themes, and, ultimately, story.

Writers must be close observers. Many—like Mark Doty, Mary Oliver, and Anne Morrow Lindbergh— have their eye trained on the natural world. This is what Elisabeth Tova Bailey does in her book, *The Sound of a Wild Snail Eating*. Like the snail she observes in a bedside terrarium, Bailey never leaves the room where she is confined because of debilitating exhaustion and weakness. Bailey not only finds comfort and companionship through her intimate observations of this small animal, she uses these observations to delve more deeply into her own situation. Here are some of Bailey's observations:

The creature seemed to defy physics. It moved over the very tips of mosses without bending them, and it could travel straight up the stem of a fern and then continue upside down along the frond's underside... Its balance, too, was impeccable. It could perch on the very edge of the mussel shell and from this precarious position reach casually across to open space to eat some of the mushrooms without falling or spilling water from the shell... Each morning the terrarium glistened with the silvery trails of its nighttime travels...

Several times I was lucky enough to see it grooming; it arched its neck over the curved edge of its own shell and cleaned the rim carefully with its mouth, like a cat licking fur on the back of its neck. Usually the snail slept on its side, and at those times the striae, perpendicular to the spiraling whorls of its shell, reminded me of the pattern of stripes on my old tiger cat, Zephyr, when he would curl into a nap.

And here are some of the connections Bailey made:

My own adventures were more challenging. After weeks of never leaving the bed in the room where I stayed, a trip to a doctor's appointment was a monumental undertaking. I traveled horizontally in the car, and given the physical stillness of my usual daily existence, it was astonishing to see the treetops rushing past overhead at what seemed like a furious speed.

Unlike the sturdy external shell of my snail, my supporting structure was internal. But the bones that made up the skeleton deep within me were losing their density at a rapid rate, and there was little I or my doctors could do to halt the problem. My status as a vertebrate was literally dissolving. I would eventually become a spineless, soft-bodied creature, more like a gastropod than a mammal. And unless my armpits could secrete shell material, I would be more slug- than snail-like.

Writing Prompt

- Pick an object at random. Don't think about your choice or specifically seek out an object with meaning. The point of this exercise is to let the object lead you, not vice versa. Now study your object. View it from all sides. If it isn't too heavy, hold it in your hands and feel its weight. Close your eyes and run your hands over the object. Note its texture, temperature, edges, rounded surfaces. Think of the fable about the blind men who each come up with a very different description of an elephant depending upon which part of the body they are describing—an ear, a tusk, a leg, etc. Do this with your object, describing only one section at a time, thinking of ways you could name it with only this partial information. Does your object have any parts that move or that shift? Does it have a smell? What sound does it make if you knock it with your knuckles, with a spoon? What are the metaphors that the object inspires in you? Write all of your observations.

Begin to make associations with what you discover about the object and the larger thoughts your study might have triggered. Is there some quality or association you have made that might be a jumping-off point for writing about your state of mind or state of being? How can the object help you to tell a piece of your story?

You can do this exercise as many times as you want. You don't have to limit yourself to man-made items—a tree, a leaf, a flower, an acorn, a cloud, a sunset, etc., would also work.

• Writing about personal experience requires close observation of the past. Pick a house you used to live in, your childhood bedroom, a classroom, or the house of worship you attended, and describe the physical layout of the place as well as the smells, the sounds, the lighting, what happened there, the people, the mood, etc.

Listen Closely: A Warm-Up For Your Ears

Dialogue can help you to show, rather than tell, your story. Through the words of your characters you can create a deeper picture of the personalities in your story, move the action forward, create mood, and find interesting ways to weave in some of your back story. Writing dialogue begins with listening. Listen to the way people speak—not just their words but their rhythm, cadence, colloquialisms, tone—to make dialogue authentic. That includes paying attention to your own voice, as well.

Paying attention is a polite way of saying eavesdropping. Maybe you find yourself at a restaurant and you are drawn in by the conversation between two women, one of whom is struggling with the best way to care for an ailing mother. You whip out your notebook and, in good stenographic fashion, create a verbatim transcription of their conversation. You think you have great material for your story, and you do, somewhere amid the interruptions of the wait staff, the ping of a text message, comments about the food, and maybe a little gossip about an acquaintance sitting across the room. Reading your transcription back you think, *no one actually speaks like this, with so many repetitions, redundancies, incomplete sentences, dropped thoughts, pauses and stutters.* But this is precisely how we speak, it just doesn't make for very good reading.

The job of the writer is similar to that of a chef who, to make a rich sauce, must boil down her ingredients to get rid of excess liquid and leave only the flavor. You leave out the parts about ordering iced tea and wondering if Miss X in the corner had a nose job. "Ums" and "uhs" that are merely space fillers can be deleted, as can the multiple times we often begin our story again after interruptions. What you are left with is the central narrative—about the mother who insists on living alone, who gets up at night because she thought she heard a sound downstairs, who slips on that damn area rug at the top of the stairs, who ends up with a concussion and bruised ribs, who is making her daughter feel helpless because she doesn't know what to do. While you are listening you are also watching so you can include the exhales, the bowed heads, the eye contact between friends, the attempts at a smile.

Writing Prompt

- Take your notebook and go out and eavesdrop. Write down what you hear. Also, take notes about gestures, expressions, attire, tics, etc. Once you have your conversation, rewrite it so it is distilled to its essence.

- Get to know your own voice. Write a conversation from memory. It could be of a fight you had, a confession you made, the time you introduced your boyfriend or girlfriend to your parents, etc. Write honestly; if you said something you regret or that was hurtful, don't flinch from writing it down. We write not to exonerate ourselves, but to know who we are.

Change Your Seat

It is a humid day in mid-August. Nadia, age four, and I go to the beach with pails and shovels ready to construct something great. The sky is a pastel blue as the light filters through the thick air. Our eyes squint against the sparkle of sun on ocean. We fill buckets with sand and upend them to form our castle walls, we create roads and dig canals that fill with water. I am engrossed in our project and in Nadia. I shift my direction from east to west to start a new section and look up. Black thunderclouds create a completely new vista and mood. Even as the sun still shines on my back, the coming storm in front of me changes me from playmate to mother. I grab Nadia and our supplies and run back toward the house.

Changing our seat, a phrase taken from Rabbi David Ingber's thoughts on moving from judgment to compassion, is what we, as storytellers, must do. One of the biggest risks we take in writing memoir is hurting a friend's or loved-one's feelings. Or, as we write about those who have, or we think have, hurt or angered us, we spread our ill feelings onto the page, threatening to poison our story with vitriol. We want to write the truth, but we must do so by looking at what has happened to us from multiple viewpoints.

For years in my journal I wrote about my husband as if he were simply an adjunct to our family. Each entry supported the truth that I was the primary caregiver, that my husband thought it was enough to swoop in to play with the kids once in a while, that the real child-rearing part was done by me. It was a very whiny journal, boring even me after a while. What was missing was any understanding of my husband's love of being a parent. If he wasn't home because he had to work so hard, it was to create a safe haven for his family. If he disrupted the bath schedule with his high energy, I could have chosen to join in the fun rather than resent this disruption to the routine. Instead of ignoring or not seeking his parenting advice, I could have remembered that one reason I married him was because of his values. When Nadia was sick I thought my pain was so much worse than my husband's because I was the caregiver, as if that meant I loved Nadia more, that I felt more pain and sorrow. I had to swivel in my chair to see the elements that challenged my assumptions. Now I could hold two truths; yes, I was the primary caregiver and that made me feel as if I was being given too much of a burden at times, and yes, I could find solace in the fact that my husband loved Nadia and it was often my assumption of all control that kept him from doing more.

Writing Prompt

- Move your seat, literally. If you always sit in the same place at the dinner table, in a class, at the movies, on your couch, the same bench in the park, etc., move your position. Write about what is different. It may not just be the view. It could be that you see new facial expressions among the people you are with, or maybe you notice someone you never have before. The new view could change your mood—perhaps it is less pretty or darker. You might hear different sounds in your new seat. Even your posture might be different.

- Make a list of the hurts and angers that you are holding on to and the circumstances or people that gave rise to them. Pretend they are holograms that you can circle around. As your perspective changes, what new truths can you find? Does holding more than one view enable you to be more compassionate?

- Write about a time you changed your mind. One example for me was choosing to use humor when I realized that the seriousness with which I had been speaking to Nadia would not help her cope with losing her hair.

List Making

We all create lists. We keep running tallies of what we need at the grocery store, what we must pack for a trip, who we have to invite to a birthday party, questions we have for a doctor. We write them on scraps, in organizers, on pads in the kitchen. Lists can give us a feeling of control. We write something down and it is the same as having an action plan; buy milk, pack a warm sweater, invite the new kid to the party, and we can go to sleep feeling secure that the day went as we expected. But lists can also be our tormentors, taunting us with all we have to do, questions that have no answers, goals we may never reach.

When woven into our writing, lists can help set a scene, convey what is overwhelming us, add a rush of forward motion to the narrative. They are a catalog, evidence of who we are, our values, our desires, our needs.

Tim O'Brien wrote his semiautobiographical novel *The Things They Carried* as a way of grappling with his experience in the Vietnam War. There is a close correlation between writing about illness and writing about war. In both cases, we write to understand and to heal, both emotionally and physically. This book was not O'Brien's first attempt at writing on the subject of war. In searching for a new way, he turns, in the first chapter, to lists. Indeed, this chapter is the quintessential example of how lists can create power, define personalities, and make the lives of a group of soldiers in Vietnam real for a reader who has never been in a war.

> *The things they carried were largely determined by necessity. Among the necessities were P-38 can openers, pocket knives, heat tabs, wristwatches, dog tags, mosquito repellent, chewing gum, candy, cigarettes, salt tablets, packets of Kool-Aid, lighters, matches, sewing kits, Military Payment Certificates, C-rations, and two or three canteens of water.*

O'Brien differentiates his characters by what they carry. The list for the medic includes not just first aid supplies but M&M's. One man carries a photo, another his girlfriend's stocking, another tranquilizers. He also differentiates by function—of rank, of necessity, of mission, of superstition. A list doesn't have to include physical objects. O'Brien adds these items to the list:

> *They carried all the emotional baggage of men who might die. Grief, terror, love, longing—these were intangibles, but the intangibles had their own mass and specific gravity, they had tangible weight. They carried shameful memories. They carried the common secret of cowardice...*

Writing Prompt

- Play with making lists to tell a story, paint a portrait, set a scene or a mood. Some suggestions include:

Things you carry

Steps you take to get ready to go out

Questions for the doctor

Directions on how to assemble something, get somewhere, prepare a meal, cure an illness

Gifts that people have given you

People who come to visit

Tests/Procedures/Medications

Music playlists

Steps of a ritual

What's in your closet, pocketbook, briefcase, sewing box, garage, tool kit, junk drawer, etc.

- Look back on your lists and think about what you would have written five, ten, fifteen or more years ago. Create a list timeline to illustrate how your interests, tastes, and needs have changed, and/or to show what aspects of your life have remained constant.

- Pick one list and weave it into a narrative.

- If one or more items on your lists jump out at you, take some time to develop your thoughts about that one particular item.

- Are you a list-maker, are your spices lined up in a rack in alphabetical order, do you balance your checkbook each month, is your closet organized by season or color? In other words, how organized are you? Do you have systems? Do you use them?

- Read *The Things They Carried*

Text, Tweet, Haiku

A friend about to have surgery sent me the following text: "It's 3 am...I know. I can't sleep. I can hear Ayla and Feisty snoring lightly in the room." The fear and isolation of the writer is clear, mitigated at that moment only by the soft breathing of her beloved dogs. Our stories don't always need to be told in long paragraphs and with many words. Poets have a great deal to teach us about peeling and stripping and paring until you get to the precise words that tell your truth.

Many see texting and tweeting as a threat to long-form narrative. But the restrictions of these modes of communication can serve as molds for our words. We can fill the mold with sugar and air or we can blend rich dark chocolate with chopped nuts and fruit and maybe a splash of rum. We can throw our words into the wind or we can write with the sensibility of a poet, laying down phrases that will sink into the reader's heart.

A form of poetry that Twitter is made for is haiku. It should be no surprise that there is even a TwiHaiku.com website. The traditional haiku is seventeen syllables divided into three lines of five-seven-five. This rule is now more of a guideline. The main feature of a haiku is the juxtaposition of two ideas through the sharing of a brief moment.

Rereading the journal I kept during Nadia's treatment, I underlined certain passages that returned me to the exact moment they depicted. As an exercise, I went through these entries and condensed them into haiku poems. It was an illuminating exercise. Whether I'm a good writer of haiku or not doesn't matter; what affected me as a writer was being forced to dig even deeper to understand the core of my writing. I've included a few examples here of both the original entry and the haiku.

> *What good will a brush with death do for this empathic, generous, strong, patient, and determined girl?*

Death brushes by
Choose someone else who
Can learn from you.

I don't let Nadia see me cry or witness my fear and helplessness, so how can she know how deeply I hurt for her?

Secret tears
She can't see how I
Hurt for her

I love the continuity of memories. But everything, for me, is always tinged or even darkly colored with melancholy. The memories are reminders of what will never be again. Tradition becomes a minefield when you realize that no two years are exactly the same, that you can never be certain or in control.

Feet in the past
I walk a line of memories
A melancholy minefield

Writing Prompt

- Practice writing texts, tweets, or haikus with the mindfulness of a poet. When you are out and about, pay attention to your surroundings using all five senses. What brief scenes or moments strike you—the ring of a cardinal's mating call when the snow is still a foot deep, the sound of laughter in an emergency room, a lone skier coming down the mountain for the last run of the day, the disparity between how a dish is described on a menu and what actually appears.

- Go through some of your writing and make haikus out of various sections. Return to what you originally wrote and see if, after writing the haiku, you see an opportunity for tightening your work.

- Imagine some of the more acute moments in your experience as a patient or caregiver and condense that time into a tweet or text. Create a thumbnail portrait of what you are experiencing. Imagine a group of these portraits. See what happens when you link them up to create a poem.

In the Image of a Person

We are our own strongest point of reference when searching for ways to describe an object or abstract notion—how we speak, behave, move, and appear. Personification—imbuing a concept, inanimate object, or an animal with human characteristics—peppers our speech from an early age, when dishes run away with spoons, teapots shout to pour me out, and Old Mother Hubbard's dog smokes a pipe, plays the flute, and wears clothes. We make light tiptoe, waves dance, time fly, life pass us by, and wind sing. Mythology and religious writings are filled with personification. While the lesson we are supposed to learn from the latter is that we are made in the image of a higher being, what we are actually creating, in a literary sense, is a being created in our own image.

I think we make these connections between ourselves and something "other" without conscious thought, without knowing that we are giving human attributes to an agent or phenomenon. But when we do it with purpose we can move our understanding of emotions or states of being from the general to the specific as Jane Kenyon did in this excerpt from her poem "Happiness":

No, happiness is the uncle you never
knew about, who flies a single engine plane
onto the grassy landing strip, hitchhikes
into town, and inquires at every door
until he finds you asleep midafternoon
as you so often are during the unmerciful
hours of your despair.

The thirteenth-century Persian poet and mystic known as Rumi wrote an extended poem of personification in "The Guest House," translated by Coleman Barks, which asks us to view those things that hurt us in an atypical way.

This being human is a guest-house.
Every morning a new arrival.

A joy, a depression, a meanness,
some momentary awareness comes
as an unexpected visitor.
Welcome and entertain them all!
Even if they're a crowd of sorrows,
who violently sweep your house
empty of its furniture,
still, treat each guest honorably.

He may be clearing you out
for some new delight.

The dark thought, the shame, the malice,
meet them at the door laughing,
and invite them in.

Be grateful for whoever comes,
because each has been sent
as a guide from beyond.

Writing Prompt

• Practice using personification to describe objects or thoughts. You can begin simply by looking around your environment and describing what you see. For example, I am sitting in a library now and here are a few ways I can describe the setting: Computer keys nag at my ears with their secret chatter. My chair squats and squeaks, threatening to eject me if I am too idle. Clouds, tall buildings, and shaded windows police the amount of light that enters the room. The next sentence I want to write does a taunting jig just beyond my reach. The reference books standing at attention on their shelves dare me to imagine that someday I might hold some of their knowledge. Sniffles, throat clearing, and coughs circle the room as if playing a game of telephone with each other.

Think about using personification to amplify the juxtaposition of medical paraphernalia against the familiar objects in your home. For example, the pill bottles in the medicine chest stand like children on the opposite team in red rover, red rover, blocking me from the creams and scents that used to be the mother's hands that soothed me. Personify a hospital bed, an IV pole, a scanner, a stethoscope, a syringe.

If You Were the Weather

The Perfect Storm by Sebastian Junger is filled with characters—boat captains and fishermen, lovers and mothers, coast guard rescuers and meteorologists. But the main character is the storm itself; the meeting of Hurricane Grace with two other storm systems results in a weather phenomenon so massive it becomes the story's protagonist. Writing of the captain of the *Andrea Gail's* battle with the sea, Junger observes, "...Billy's no longer at the helm, the conditions are, and all he can do is react." The storm is the force against which all the characters eventually react and respond.

Illness is a kind of weather system—a storm front that makes landfall amidst family and loved-ones, altering the environment, eroding the breakwaters we have erected that were meant to keep us from harm. And illness alters our internal weather conditions; where once we might have been a calm coastal high, suddenly we might be transformed into a high-altitude whiteout. Blowing snow pellets and the lack of oxygen make it impossible to take a deep breath. Our footprints are lost behind us and there is no way to tell which direction is forward.

Writing Prompt

- This is a two-part prompt that uses weather as metaphor to help you and others understand the illness you are dealing with, either as the patient, the caregiver, a family member, or a healer. First, write about the effect of illness on your life as if it were a weather system. Think back to the first symptoms, the day of the diagnosis, the progression, the effect of treatment. Track your "illness system" the way a meteorologist would track a weather system. Use meteorological terminology. Feel free to draw maps.

Second, picture yourself as a weather system. What meteorological phenomena reflect your emotional and physical condition right now? Unlike the real weather, yours can include contradictory elements. You can be a snowstorm in eighty-degree weather; the sky can be a perfect blue while it's pouring rain. What is the impact of your weather system on the environment (i.e., your home, place of business, family)? What happens when your weather system meets up with someone else's? Is your current state more a Yankee Clipper or a stalled front?

• Become an observer of the weather. Write about what you see, feel, and experience.

• Use the weather metaphor to write about places, i.e., a hospital room, doctor's office, your bedroom, a waiting room, a place where you go for respite, etc.

This Is How It's Done

My children all learned how to drive on a car with an automatic transmission. But on Martha's Vineyard, we have a Jeep Wrangler that the kids love; it's so much more fun to drive to the beach in a car with no roof or windows, that you can climb in and out of without opening doors, and in which your black dog, scrunched in the back seat with your friends, can raise its nose to the sky. The problem, of course, is that the Jeep has a stick shift and it was my job to teach the kids how to drive it.

I grew up driving a car with a manual transmission; it had been a long time since I had to dissect the process. The beginning lessons were easy—showing where the clutch was, which foot operated it. The kids learned how to move the stick through the gears, doing a dance with the feet between the clutch, brake, and accelerator. Then it was time to start the car. *Always be sure the clutch is depressed when you start the car. If you're in gear and you lift your foot off the clutch the car will stall.* Now it was time to move with the engine on. How do you describe the process of easing out the clutch and giving the car gas? How do you convey the feeling of the magic moment when each is in perfect balance and you can start forward in smooth acceleration? *Too much gas. Oops, not enough. Too fast on the clutch. I can't speak while I'm laughing so hard.*

By this time we had made it fifteen feet down the driveway. What could I say to help? Like so many things, it came down to the breath. *Okay, shift into first. Inhale. Now ease up on the clutch and down on the accelerator as you sigh. Aaah. Perfect.*

Describing an action that you do without thinking is a great exercise in paying attention to detail. In *Motherhood Exaggerated*, I describe the process of changing the dressing over Nadia's Broviac, the central IV line, implanted in her chest. The dressing needed to be changed three days a week because it is a breach in the body's armor and germs and bacteria must be fended off. Here is what I wrote:

> *First, remove the dressing. Open sterile kit containing supplies. Put on surgical mask so mother's germs won't poison child. Wash sweaty hands. Put on gloves. Peel off old bandage, which will pull at delicate skin and make it red, sore, and itchy. Check the site for inflammation. Throw contaminated gloves away.*

Second, clean and rebandage. Open sterile field, like an oversized napkin, touching only the edges of the paper. Put sterile gloves on shaky hands. Do not brush hair from eyes, scratch an itch, answer the phone, or touch anything outside your germ-free area until task is completed. Open the three alcohol and three blood-red Povidone swabs contained in kit. Place on sterile field with gauze and Primapore bandages. Clean site three times with alcohol that stings. Wash with Povidone. Let air dry. Be sure that child doesn't breathe on site, dogs don't come over to play, and siblings stay far away with their sneezes and coughs. Cover with gauze, then bandages. Remove mask made damp from nervous breaths. Sigh deeply.

Third, secure the tubes. Loop and tape tubes to chest so they don't hang and pull. Attach to undershirt with safety pin showing so next time you have to change the dressing, you won't whip the shirt off with the tubes still attached and cause unbearable pain to child. Throw garbage away. Resume living.

Writing Prompt

- Describe something that you do every day as if you were telling someone who would have to imitate you. It could be brushing your teeth (dragging yourself out of bed, shuffling to the bathroom, the cold tiles on your feet, getting out supplies, running the water, the foam of the toothpaste making you gag, the movement of the brush, the faces you make, what you are thinking about, staring at your face in the mirror, etc.), washing your hair, making a grilled cheese sandwich, applying makeup, making a bed, fixing a perfect martini, etc.

- Repeat the above exercise, but show yourself in various moods. How do your actions change when you are angry, sad, newly in love, etc.?

- Now, write a similar description of an action or activity that flows from the experience of illness. It could be learning to walk in a physical therapy session, getting dressed, taking medications, having a test or scan done, changing into a hospital gown, preparing special food, etc.

A Hand Portrait

I have always been fascinated with hands. People who have had plastic surgery end up with faces whose stories have been erased, with tummies that no longer show evidence of the lip-smacking meals they digested, and with breasts upon which it would seem no baby ever nursed. Hands, though, continue to tell a story all through life. My mother's hands had the heft and authenticity of sterling silver. But during her depression when I was a teenager, the steeple formed by her fingers became as porous as an ancient church ruin. Alzheimer's made my father's hands restless like two spiders that couldn't figure out where to build their webs. Here is a study of my own hands.

> *There are creases in the palms of my hand. Not the lines of life, head, heart, or fate that are supposed to tell me my destiny. No, these creases are the ones caused by gripping. They are the row of small arcs made by my nails which I see when I uncurl my fists in the morning; they are the ridges on my thumb from clenching my pencil when I write; they are the indentations made by the book that I hold too close to my face. They*

come from gripping the steering wheel, the weights in the gym, cups of tea, knitting needles, and my watch, which I twist and fiddle with as if it weren't a keeper of time but of a place between moments.

My fingers clenched around syringes—some containing the fertility drugs I said I would try just once, some holding the epinephrine I had to inject into my son when he had an anaphylactic reaction to food, some holding the white-blood-cell–building serum to inject into my younger daughter after her rounds of chemotherapy. I grabbed for my older daughter who injected lightness into these moments.

I gripped my babies until they gripped back too hard, making it difficult for us to release each other when I needed my hands to hold more than another person's future.

The skin on my hands no longer clings tightly to bone. Pinch a piece of flesh and it takes longer to lie flat. I try to see those blood-filled, raised veins as symbols of strength and experience, but if I stare too long I can feel the blood rushing and swelling and I have to hold my hands above my head to staunch the tide.

Sometimes I remember not to clench. I stretch my fingers wide; they span just short of an octave on the piano. I imagine the space between my joints filling with air. As my hands relax my jaw clenches. I relax my mouth and my fingers start to curl toward my palms. A part of me always needs to hold on, but the only thing I can find to grip is myself.

Writing Prompt

- Study your own hands. Look at your nails, the creases around your knuckles, the length of your fingers, age spots, veins, and scars. Run your hands against each other. Where are the rough spots? The areas that have remained protected? Close your eyes and think about the gestures you make when you talk, how you hold a pencil, the nervous way they keep touching your hair or tapping the table. Now, create a self-portrait by writing about your hands. In addition to what you see, write about what your hands used to do and what they do now; what they touch, stroke, slap, create, pull toward you, or push away; what makes them shake or sweat; show your hands when they are angry, nervous, impatient, sad, laughing, dancing, sleeping, bored. What about rings—do you wear them, do they tell a story, do they still fit? Do your hands hold the hands of others, who holds yours, etc.

- Try this same exercise using other parts of your body.

- Write about someone else's hands as they interact with yours.

Part II

Parting the Curtains, Setting the Scenes

This section asks you to delve into your story of illness. It takes courage to bring yourself back to moments of pain—emotional, physical, or both. The act of writing, as opposed to talking, about even the most difficult experiences will give you distance. But when you read back what you have written you will find that the pain has made it onto the page. As writers, we also have the option of writing in the third person. Even though we know we are telling our own story, replacing each "I" with "he/she" automatically gives us the ability to stand a bit apart from what we are saying. Be sure you take care of yourself during this process. Don't flinch from what is hard, but give yourself breaks and rewards as you go along.

Writing these scenes also requires that we pay very close attention to the details, a skill I hope you had a chance to practice in the previous section. You want to bring yourself (and any future reader, if you plan on sharing your work) into the sights, sounds, smells, and sensations of the moment. Remember this as you begin to write, particularly if you are having a hard time getting started. Your scenes will be vivid and vibrant.

This is also the place where the pace of your journey can slow down. Sit and watch the scene unfolding in your mind before moving onto another one. This is harder than it sounds. Once you get started, memories and feelings will begin to percolate. Make a quick note of these on a piece of paper if you are worried about forgetting them, but return to the present scene you are observing in your mind's eye. If you meditate, this instruction will sound very familiar.

Each chapter offers a number of different writing suggestions. Do the ones that make the most sense to you at any particular moment. As your story starts to unfold, you may find yourself returning to previous chapters to explore new territory. You may jump ahead, or you may find you can put the book aside for a while as your words flow on their own.

It is up to you whether you want to write individual moments and small pieces, more extended personal essays, or a longer-form memoir. These exercises will give you the option to do any of these. Write freely. That means writing beautifully and badly, making no sense and then finding wisdom. Give your inner critic a name and tell him or her to be quiet. Once you have finished writing and you want to create a more polished piece you will find tips on revision at the end of this book.

Now imagine the sound of a soft chime and begin.

When You Found Out

"There is a before. And there is the forever after.
And
There
Is
The
Frozen
Moment
that marks the rent in a family's life, the stygian
introduction to the new, upside-down world that
they are about to enter when they first hear the
words, 'Your daughter has cancer'."

These are the opening words of Dr. Leonard Wexler's foreword to my first book, *Motherhood Exaggerated*. He is right. When he told my husband and me that our daughter had cancer we were sent into a place of darkness. But when I think back to that period of discovery and diagnosis, break it down into minutes and hours rather than viewing it as a single block of time, it is easy to see that the darkness didn't so much descend as creep closer, swirl around us, and then, with the final pronouncement, envelop us.

There was no moment when we didn't know and then we did. Symptoms and preliminary tests scattered clues like bread crumbs, ones that at first seemed randomly placed, then ones whose trail we were loath to follow, then ones that pulled us along like a moving sidewalk with no off-ramp. The final declaration, that Nadia had a Ewing's sarcoma, came after the biopsy, which showed she had cancer but not what kind; which came after the most likely diagnosis of osteogenic sarcoma; which came after "we're ninety-nine percent sure it's nothing," following the cracking of Nadia's jaw; which came after the mysterious fevers, strange humming, and Nadia's growing malaise.

What threw us into that stygian universe was the shadow cast by the words of the diagnosis over our trail of bread crumbs. Indeed, it was here that the trail ended. Finding our way back would require taking a new, unmarked route with no familiar landmarks or lampposts.

Writing Prompt

• Write about your before and after. If it is helpful, think about a door. What lies on one side of the door; what on the other? What did it feel like as you opened the door and stepped through—did it squeak on rusty hinges or glide with ease, did you trip over the threshold, did you have to be dragged, or did you run? What was the sensation when the door closed behind you? Did it lock or did it remain porous, was there a window through which you could see but not touch your former life or was what existed on the other side obliterated?

Set concrete scenes. Where were you when the words of the diagnosis were spoken? What kind of details did your mind travel to—the dust in the corner, a pair of latex gloves in the wastebasket, the sock that has fallen around the doctor's ankle. If you were at home, explore the incongruity of the conversation you are having— maybe over the phone—amongst your familiar objects and spaces. Write the conversation. Include your inner dialogue, the feelings you didn't express, the questions you didn't ask. Who else was in the room? Perhaps, if the diagnosis involved a child, you were the one who had to deliver the news. Write that conversation, how you chose your words, the questions your child asked.

Expand the reach of your senses. Contrast what was happening in your corner of experience with what might have been going on in the outside world. What noises from the street or the neighbors did you hear? What can you imagine other people were doing at the same time you were having your conversation? What would you have been doing on a typical day at this time?

•   Write about other moments when your life had to pivot, when there was a before and an after. It can be a moment from childhood, school, parenthood, a time when you moved, lost a job or was hired for a new one, fell in lust or love, etc.

Waiting

Illness is a waiting room. It punches holes in hours, days, and weeks. You wait to see or be seen, to tell or be told; for the phone to ring, the pain to arrive, the relief to start. Nearly every moment of action is preceded by waiting—not to be confused with inaction. Waiting is a very busy verb.

A story that included every moment of waiting would look moth-eaten, shredded to a point that it would disintegrate. While I waited with Nadia, or as she underwent a test or surgery where I couldn't be present, I found my thoughts focused on one of two themes. The first was the growing separation between Nadia and me in terms of what we were experiencing. Waiting for Nadia to complete her first diagnostic test, a Panorex of her jaw, I recognized that this was the point our lives began to diverge. I was waiting; she was not, at least not until the test was over when we waited for different things—me for the results, her to go home. And there was the period of time when I had knowledge but had to wait to tell Nadia because my knowledge was still incomplete. During that time, all I wanted was to bombard Nadia with the same terms I was given—

cancer, round blue cells, toxic chemotherapy—and to make her a partner in my despair. Of course, I did none of that.

The second theme waiting helped me to explore was my own helplessness. On the day of her biopsy, when Nadia was taken into the operating room, I was left outside and suspended, like being in an airport waiting area when you know there is a good chance that the plane you can't avoid boarding is going to crash. When treatment started, I waited for Nadia's counts to go up, her hair to fall out, her fever to rise, for her to explode from some catastrophic malfunction. And after treatment I waited for her to live.

Waiting rooms could give a writer material for life. They are filled with the mundane—the perpetual drone of CNN, old copies of *People, Woman's Day, AARP The Magazine, Reader's Digest.* People knit, fill out forms, try to stay connected to the outside world with phones and iPads. But the waiting room always wins. The mundane lifts away and the purpose of this holding space is revealed.

Writing Prompt

• Write about an experience of waiting. Set the external scene. Maybe you are in one room or maybe you are carrying your wait with you, from the car to the kitchen to the bath. Next, write about the physical experience—your shallow breaths, your shaky fingers trying to turn the page of a magazine, how often you shift or fidget or get up to go to the bathroom even though you don't have to go because you have to do something with waiting's unique cocktail of energy, anxiety, and boredom. Are you alone? How does that feel? If you aren't alone, show the interaction with your companion; weave a duet between what you are saying aloud with your internal dialogue. How does it feel when the wait is over—when the phone rings, your name or the name of the person you are caring for is called, the nurse comes to tell you you can see your loved-one in the recovery room? You can do this exercise often with additional experiences of waiting.

•   Pick someone who is in a waiting room with you, someone who perhaps seems new or in need of support. What would you say to that person? What would you want to ask someone else? Does anyone look as if they could be a potential friend? Would you want to make friends here?

•   Design a better waiting room. You can do this either in words or by creating a floor plan. Identify issues that are important to you such as privacy, lighting, seating, entertainment, temperature, color scheme, technology, etc. If you wish, look through magazines and cut out examples of furniture and fixtures you would want.

Why or Why Not

"Why not?" It's how I answered Nadia when she asked me why she got cancer. It sounds like such a cruel response, as if to strip her of the specialness every child is entitled to feel, especially in the eyes of their mothers. But what I wanted her to know was that she hadn't done anything to deserve her disease. There are those who might have told her otherwise. There is an organization called Chai Lifeline that provides support to Jewish families with seriously ill children. In their packet of material is a book of prayers and psalms introduced with the words: "One should recognize that all human misfortune or illness is a direct result of man's evil ways. This awareness will lead him to repentance which is an important factor in alleviating misfortune and illness." Not much of a lifeline in that for an eight-year-old girl. Not all Jews believe this way, but most religions contain some doctrine that equates illness or tragedy with either being deserved or having some higher purpose.

It is not necessary to believe in God to search for the "why" of an illness. Self-blame is its own religion. I wondered if the fertility drugs I took caused Nadia's cancer. Did the fetus that didn't survive and was reabsorbed by my body make it into Nadia's instead? Why didn't I respond earlier to the clues that Nadia was ill, even though they made sense only in retrospect? And, of course, the question that still echoes, shouldn't it have been me?

When Nadia finished her treatment, still searching for the reason she got cancer, she said, "I think God gave me cancer because He knew I was strong." The idea made me cringe. It sounded to me no different than the people who tried to tell me that God never gave us more than we can bear. Even so, I was glad Nadia saw herself as strong.

Eight years later, when Nadia had to write her college essay, she tackled the question yet again. She wrote that neither science nor religion can say why she got cancer. Science can say how and it can develop cures, religion can provide comfort. But neither will tell you why.

In his book *When Bad Things Happen To Good People,* Rabbi Harold S. Kushner asks, "Can you accept the idea that some things happen for no reason, that there is randomness in the universe?" I would rephrase this by asking, what were the questions that came after "Why?"

Writing Prompt

- When you or your loved-one received a diagnosis, suffered a trauma, or lost a family member, what were the questions that you asked? Begin with why and then continue listing questions in a stream-of-consciousness fashion. See where your questions take you. Are you still asking? Do you have an answer?

Here are my questions:

Why?

Why not?

Who are you to tell me?

How do you know?

Who should I be angry at?

Am I angry?

Why are you so angry?

What do I do now?

Can I do it?

What do I need?

Who do I tell?

What's my sister's phone number?

Should Nadia see me cry?

Where's the Tylenol?

Does Nadia still trust me?

Are we done?

Who saved Nadia's life?

Is there a point?

• Write about a turning point or time of confusion, from before illness or caregiving. What were the questions you asked yourself then? What were the values or beliefs that helped you through this time? Were you more cynical then or less, more inclined to turn toward God or away, seek community or become isolated? Has illness altered your way of responding to life's pivots? Has it changed how you respond to the question of why?

Naming an Illness

My meditation teacher tells me that, whenever negative forces or thoughts arise, I should give them a name— Anna, Rachel, Sue, etc.—as a way of neutralizing them. At first I thought giving a name to something so negative would exaggerate it, give it a legitimacy I thought it shouldn't have. But it's easier to talk to people than to feelings and talking can reduce the sting. Grief, for example, is an impenetrable block; Greta, though, is a woman with a soft voice, long hair shading her eyes, a slight limp; she is more comfortable in water than on land. I can lean into Greta to hear her speak, brush the hair from her eyes, take her hand, and guide her to the rocking waters of the sea.

Anxiety is the character I meet most often. Her name is Sybil. She greets me with a stutter. I have known her for over forty years and she has changed. Her body is still made up of the same sharp angles. Her feet still pace as if they never need sleep, my heartbeat mirroring their uneven rhythm. She still takes me by the arm, whispers in my ear of things only her silver eyes can see. But it no longer takes as much strength for me to loosen her grip, and if I whisper "shh" back to her she will become silent. Her hair, once black, spiky, and uncombed is now nearly white and contained by a headband. I don't know where Sibyl lives or the path she takes to find me. I used to make her welcome; she loves a strong cup of Irish Breakfast tea. These days I'm more inclined to stroke her long fingers, straightening and lengthening them before they can turn into claws.

Siddhartha Mukherjee, in *The Emperor of All Maladies: A Biography of Cancer*, says, "To name an illness is to describe a certain condition of suffering—a literary act before it becomes a medical one." The true literary act, though, is in the renaming of the illness, to give it a moniker that is uniquely yours. This name is not the same as your diagnosis. Many people share that label. Rather, it is an identifier of the nature and personality of what is afflicting *you*. It is a way to address your illness in familiar terms and to communicate what you are experiencing to others in a metaphorical form they can understand.

Writing Prompt

- Write about your illness as if it were a person. What name does it have? Is it male or female, and why? What does it look like—height, hair and eye color, skin tone, clothes, hands? Describe its mannerisms, habits, and moods. How does it speak? Create a dialogue between you and this character. When you are done, think about how, if at all, naming your illness this way has influenced your relationship to it.

- Caregivers and family members can do the same exercise by developing their own character based upon how they interact with their loved-one's illness. It might be interesting to compare the characters each has created, but that is strictly a personal decision because you, the writer, has to write first, and perhaps only, for your own eyes.

- Give a name and character to a feeling or emotion, i.e., pain, grief, joy, loneliness, relief, etc.

- In *Heaven's Coast*, Mark Doty tries to figure out where he is emotionally after the death of his lover. He asks "…but where was I then? Some vague lunar place, a winter shore lit only by starlight, an icy marsh." Name your illness after a place.

- If you have read *The Golden Compass* by Philip Pullman, you will know that each character has his or her own dæmon, a soul in the form of an animal. This dæmon changes during childhood but becomes fixed as the person matures. Which animal best represents your soul? Is it different than the one you would have chosen before your life was altered by illness?

Writing It Raw

The page is a vessel into which I deposit my sorrow and express my fear and confusion. Sometimes I just need to throw my words on the page. *Splat!* "I, I, I, I…" "No, no, no, no…" "You, you, you, you…" "How, how, how, how…" "Can't, can't, can't, can't…" No holding back, no filter, no reflection.

Writing is like entering a room with a whacky thermostat. My early writing about my mother was always pouty and whiny. *My mother loved my sister more than me*, I'd write. *She didn't spoil me when I was sick, leaving me alone with a throbbing head or a high temperature. She kept too many secrets from me.* As I moved through my thirties, forties, and fifties the narrative never changed. My words had stuck where I had thrown them like overdone spaghetti. I tried pouring cold water over them by pretending none of this mattered now. But it did. It affected how I raised my children, the amount of pride I felt in myself, how I held myself aloof from my husband's worries. It was only when I went beyond my own story and began to tell my mother's that my emotions found an equilibrium. Anger was replaced by compassion and compassion allowed me to recognize how much my mother loved me.

In *The Still Point of the Turning World* Emily Rapp notes that writers who move beyond what they address to their journal have gone back "...and shaped their words. They did the work of revision. They wrestled with language and form." I would add that they also wrestled with themselves.

Writing Prompt

• This is your chance to howl, to scream at the page. Remove all filters, take a deep breath, and let go. No one will hear you. Write all the harsh, intimate, angry, wrenching thoughts that travel through you. Take aim at doctors, nurses, family members, yourself, caregivers, the intrusive neighbor, the insurance representative, the insensitive person in line at the grocery store. Write about watching someone suffer, about feeling alone, about looking for someone to blame. Maybe you picked a fight with someone you loved or shut someone out. Reenact scenes that stirred your strongest emotions.

• Now, pick one of your scenes and reflect on it. How can you imbue it with compassion? What is compassion? *The Merriam-Webster Dictionary* describes it as "a sympathetic consciousness of others' distress together with a desire to alleviate it." But how do you arrive at that consciousness? Rabbi David Ingber offers, I think, a deeper definition. Compassion, he says, is holding as many sides of the truth as we can hold. In other words, you don't have to let go of what is making you tremble, but see if you can include in your writing the story of the person or circumstance you are railing against.

- One strategy might be to write the scene from another person's perspective. Another might be to place yourself as the compassionate observer and write the scene in the third person. Instead of saying "I" say, "He/she." Even though you are still writing about yourself, the third-person perspective automatically gives you a sense of distance.

- Some of what arose within you will always be too hard or too intimate or too invasive. Not everything has to go into your story. Recognize what is meant to share and what is meant only for the unread or shredded page, the soundproof room, the pillow that is the recipient of your tears.

- Create a compassionate portrait of someone who has angered or disappointed you.

- Write an apology to someone you have hurt.

Domes of Words

Where are the words that are spoken by the bedsides of patients in the hospital? I imagine that over each one of those beds is a dome made up of the conversations between mothers and fathers, doctors and family members, spouses and children. Some beds may have a string of words rising from the bed into the dome, but this line is less dense and ornate than the tangle of sentences that is woven over the patients' heads.

My husband and I began weaving our dome of words—an upside-down nest really, that didn't cup Nadia but spilled her out below us—from the moment of her diagnosis. We whispered over her head the details of her treatment. I delivered reports of doctor visits while John asked, "What does that mean?" and, "How is she feeling?" I answered as if Nadia had deputized me. She hadn't. We knew Nadia wasn't sleeping during these conversations. Still, we were surprised each time she interrupted us to say, "Stop talking about me!" Did we think because she was sick she had become deaf and dumb? Was it because she was a child that we acted as if she had no voice? Was it easier to speculate how she was feeling rather than ask her? Did we think we were protecting her?

Nadia had become sick Nadia, and sick Nadia had somehow become less the owner of her own space, the way illness made her less the owner of her body. Who was I to think that that space was mine? Not only did I bring my words into her space; I brought friends, whom Nadia asked to go away; I brought my food, which made Nadia's chemo-infused stomach turn; I brought my false cheer, my I-know-what's-good-for-you attitude.

Writing Prompt

- Write the conversations that were woven around and above you. Did you ever try to say anything? Were these conversations ever comforting—like a womb made of the soft murmurs of favorite voices?

Were you the one having the conversations over the bed of a patient? Write the dialogue. Were you aware of what you were doing? What was your reaction if the person you were talking around spoke up?

Your scenes don't have to be in a hospital. They could be in the car, a waiting room, or a dinner table. It could be a telephone conversation where one person is automatically isolated. It could be at a meeting with a member of the clergy.

- Write about a time beyond or before illness when you were made to feel marginal or excluded—perhaps by a parent or teacher, maybe by friends who seemed to know things you didn't. See if you recognize any patterns in your own behavior and response that might have had bearing on your experience as a patient or caregiver.

Where Do I Stand By the Bed

It was time to disconnect my Aunt Essie from the machines that were helping her feign life. Nine of us were gathered, including Essie's daughter Miriam. As we waited for the doctor, we engaged in a restless choreography—forming in clusters in Essie's cluttered room, pacing the hallways when Miriam asked for time alone with her mother, leaning against walls, sitting with eyes staring sightless, or with heads lowered into palms, making unnecessary trips to the bathroom or to make a phone call to sip fresher air into our lungs. When the doctor arrived to remove the breathing tube and still any alarms, the nine of us rimmed Essie's bed. My daughter Frannie ended up across from me and I went to her, leaving my Aunt Alice and my cousin Bobby alone on one side, unbalancing the raft of our grief. "What do I do now?" Miriam asked when it was all over.

Caregivers and family members are instructed in so many medical functions. During Nadia's treatment, I dispensed medicines, gave shots, suctioned her trache, cleaned the dressing around her central IV. I knew what to do if she ran a fever, felt nauseated, or became itchy from the morphine. But after her surgery to rebuild her jaw using a bone from her leg, when the tubes and catheters that protruded from her body seemed to form a barrier to my touch, there was no one to give me the steps to the dance I would have to perform for the next two weeks. Where should I stand by her bed? At her right foot and leg, which I could stroke without causing pain? At her head, where I could place my hand on her bald scalp? By her ear where I could whisper soothing words? By her side where I could hold the one hand that didn't have a peripheral IV? How was I supposed to respond to her anger? Should I flee her side when she threw whatever she could reach in frustration, or should I stay close to absorb her fury? Whom do I allow, or want, to come visit? What do I say to the sorrowful faces around me? Is that even my job, to make others feel better?

Writing Prompt

• Write about a time when the choreography of caregiving was unknown to you. What was being asked of you that you weren't sure how to provide? Did you even know what was being asked of you?

• If you were the patient, write about a time when you felt the insecurity of those around you. Describe their actions and how you responded. Did you help guide those trying to help you? Did you resent their inability to know on their own?

I Should Have Said...

When illness arrives, we have to speak words we never thought would come out of our mouths. They are scary words, with thorns and spikes. They sting our tongues as we speak them and, too often, we fail to wrap them in softness to protect the person we are directing them toward.

It is painful for me now to remember some of the ways I spoke to Nadia when I was trying to explain what was happening to her. I worried that a tone of voice that was too gentle or mirrored Nadia's confusion would feed her anxiety. I wanted to be direct, but, my words echo back to me through time as too blunt. When Nadia asked me why she got cancer, my answer was, "Why not?" Maybe I added a more soothing phrase or stroked her hair, but I never stopped to look beyond the question to what she really wanted answered, "Was it something I did wrong?"

I kept a notebook for the questions I wanted to ask the doctors but spoke off the cuff to my family. I thought I had chosen each of my words so carefully when I told Nadia she had cancer. I fashioned my sentences like a bespoke tailor. Nadia's eyes opened wide and I thought she understood, but she didn't know a tumor was cancer, she thought the central IV line implanted in her chest after the biopsy was only going to stay in for a few days, and that the only surgery she would need was one to straighten out the tooth that was knocked over by the tumor. As I brought her more and more news—none of it good—I could see her recoil whenever I opened my mouth to speak, despite learning to adapt my words to Nadia's level of understanding and accompanying them with soothing gestures.

I made no attempt to protect or mollify my husband. Why should he be shielded when I wasn't? How I spoke to him was made more complicated by the fact that I didn't know what I wanted from him, how to ask him to relieve me of the burden of being the primary caregiver that I was. I either excluded him or belittled his moments of helplessness. There are so many conversations I wish I had stripped of their barbs.

Writing Prompt

- Write about a conversation(s) you wish had gone differently. Write the original conversation and then rewrite it as if you had a do-over. As you change the words you spoke, be aware of how that changes the response of the other person.

- Has illness altered the way in which you speak to others? Think about some of the conversations you have had in a group setting—with family members, doctors, in support groups. Are there words you wish you hadn't spoken, questions you didn't ask, feelings you didn't consider, arguments you didn't make?

- Write a conversation(s) that you never had the chance to have.

I Remember, I Remember Not

"Where's your husband?" From the time I began telling stories about raising my children, that's the question I am most frequently asked. And it never changes. I write about family dinners, separation anxiety, health crises, empty nesting, and don't notice I haven't included my husband. I'm not forgetting about him; I just don't remember him—his presence, the role he played in the drama, anything he said. It's a reflection of how we both made it possible for me, as the mother, to take control.

It was no different when it came to telling the story of being a mother to a child with cancer. John was a reliable presence. I know he was there for doctors' appointments, for trips to urgent care, for scans, and evenings at home when Nadia didn't have to be in the hospital. I know we must have spoken and that he and Nadia had their own conversations. But the only moments I remember are the ones in which we disagreed or in which John became the focus of my resentment. John was part of the story, but he was not part of my story.

How can you write your story if you don't remember how the whole thing goes? It's not like a song when you can just sing la-la-la when you forget the lyrics. But no one can recall every detail, especially the farther you go back in time. Not only are the memories more distant but they are no longer raw. They have been filtered through layers of years and experiences the way an underground aquifer is filtered through dirt and sediment to reach an above-ground spring.

Frank McCourt's *Angela's Ashes* challenged all memoirists as the author recounted, word for word and step by step, the conversations and events of his childhood. These conversations could not have been exact transcripts. They were reconstituted based on McCourt's remembrance of time and tone, his ear for speech patterns, his knowledge of the people into whose mouths he put the words. This is more than the "emotional truth" that people often feel is enough to justify filling the "I don't know" spaces with an "it could have happened" scenario; for example, your doctor was incompetent but you can't remember the details exactly so you make up what happened because the means justify the end.

When pressed to include John in the story of Nadia and me, I could have come up with plausible scenarios and dialogue, but the reader would have been fooled into thinking John and I were more of a pair than we were in the care of our children. It's important to pay attention to memory lapses to see if they advance your story. In my case, observing how little I had paid attention to my husband's experience gave my ultimate transformation as a wife and mother greater depth.

When a memory lapse creates a hole in your narrative that must be bridged, you can turn to others to help recreate a moment. Susannah Cahalan did just that to write her memoir, *Brain on Fire*. Afflicted with a rare autoimmune disorder that mimicked a form of madness, Cahalan had little memory of events during the most serious stage of her illness. "Because I am physically incapable of remembering that time, writing this book has been an exercise in comprehending what was lost."

Writing Prompt

• Think of a scene or a moment in time you want to write about. Put your fingers on the keyboard or a pen to paper and write, "I remember…" Without stopping, begin the next lines with either "I remember" or "I don't remember." Keep going until you run out of steam. Don't look back on what you have written until you are all done. Now write your scene based on your list. Notice if there are any patterns.

• Find a person who experienced the same moment with you. Each of you write your own version of what happened. Compare them.

• What is your first childhood memory? What is a piece of family lore that you don't remember or remember very differently from others?

• Write about what you want to forget.

• Write an elegy or an ode to someone based upon your memories of him or her.

Travelogue of Illness

> *The first trip to the Memorial Sloan-Kettering Cancer Center is like arriving anywhere new. A plane takes you down through thick clouds, a train moves you through a dark tunnel, a bus pulls up to the rear of a terminal while you paint images in your head of this foreign land soon to be revealed... We are the pale new arrivals at the beachside resort, catching a glimpse of a sliver of its life.*

This is how I described taking Nadia to the Memorial Sloan-Kettering Cancer Center for the first time.

Without making a conscious decision to equate illness with a physical place one arrives at and journeys through, I found the vocabulary of travel apt. I hesitated when it came to comparing a medical center to a resort, worried that it would minimize the horror of bringing my eight-year-old daughter to a cancer hospital. But I couldn't escape the sensation that we were entering as exotic a world as any unknown vacation or adventure destination. MSKCC was a mutant Brigadoon, a place you see only when you take a trip there.

The travel metaphor is used by many writers to describe the experience of illness. Anatole Broyard, in *Intoxicated by My Illness*, describes his prostate cancer as "… a visit to a disturbed country, rather like contemporary China." In *Autobiography of a Face*, Lucy Grealy observes, "Suddenly I understood the term visiting. I was in one place, they were in another and they were only pausing."

In his introduction to *The Tao of Travel*, Paul Theroux says, "The travel narrative is the oldest in the world, the story the wanderer tells to the folk gathered around the fire after his or her return from a journey." Journey, of course, means more than a trip to a distant geography. The listener is not as interested in what the traveler packed in his or her suitcase (although a sidebar is always helpful), but what is carried within that person—the reason for the trip, what or who is being left behind or coming with; does the narrator have a hearty appetite for adventure, a delicate stomach, claustrophobia, a sense of humor, frequent-flyer miles, many friends or a chosen few, a need for high thread-count sheets? It is the emotional and transformational souvenirs that the storyteller returns with that keep listeners around the fire, that equip them for going to that place themselves.

Whether you are a patient, a family member, or a caregiver, you are traveling a new path. You are entering a new culture, hearing new languages, encountering different norms of behavior, negotiating a new topography and geography.

Writing Prompt

- Write a travelogue of your journey. Use all of your senses to bring the reader into the same space in which you find yourself, in the same way you would describe a city street scene, a seaside boardwalk, or a hike on the Appalachian Trail. For example, you can write about the hospital as a foreign country—what are the rules about entering, who lives/works/visits there, what language is spoken, how do you travel there, what do you bring and wear, how does it feel to inhale the air, what is the food like? Or the place can be your home. You didn't travel there, but imagine you lived in Russia when it became the Soviet Union. You are now in a new country with new norms and rules. What would you say about this new country you live in so the reader can understand what has happened to you? You could place yourself in school or the workplace or a visit to your hometown for a Thanksgiving family reunion. Take photographs to accompany your travelogue, draw pictures, add recipes of the "local" cuisine, and, yes, say what you have packed—in the suitcase you carry and in your heart.

- Tell your story by using your body as your landscape. How has its terrain changed? Does it still feel like a familiar place where you are comfortable living or does it feel like a new country you must get used to?

- Are you an enthusiastic or reluctant traveler? Write about your relationship with travel. Can you travel now? Where would or do you go?

We Are Family

Three days after Nadia's surgery, I still hadn't slept more than an hour or two each night. On a rainy afternoon, Nadia drifts into sleep. The hospital hallway is quiet. No alarm bells are ringing. I put up the footrest on my sleeper-chair and close my eyes. My breaths come deeper, sleep beckons. Knock, knock. It's a quiet tapping but feels like a shout. It is my father. I sigh. I have found no role for him to play in this drama. A quiet man, he would have had a purpose if he could have taken Nadia for a hike in his woods in New Hampshire or built something with her at his workbench. As it was, his only role was to look on. He was unable to disguise his sadness, which I felt the need to salve, even when my need felt so much greater than his.

Another scene. It is the week before Nadia's surgery. I have decided to make a poster for her hospital room; a collage filled with photographs of a strong and healthy Nadia, of family members, of school friends. Frannie decides she wants to make one, too. I tell her she can't. "This is my idea," I say. I enjoy the idea of doing something creative for Nadia. Frannie designs her own project. She makes Popsicle-stick figures with magazine cutouts, using the legs from one person, the torso from another, the head of a third. Nadia loves them; even with her swollen face and wired jaw, you can see the merriment in her eyes. Only Frannie is able to lift Nadia not just from her pain but from her boredom with me, whom she needs but with whom she can't just be a kid and do kid things. Perhaps to Frannie's detriment, I often made her my surrogate. Still, I felt incompetent when Nadia would cry, "Where's Frannie? I want Frannie."

Family. These people—our parents, spouses, siblings, children, cousins, aunts, uncles, in-laws and steps, greats and grands—are often the reason we are compelled to write, to enter therapy, to choose where we live, what rituals we observe, what brand of toothpaste we buy, what our cell phone plan should be.

During illness, we are at our most vulnerable and, therefore, most aware of the way family supports and fails us. Sometimes the two ends of the spectrum appear the same, as if they have bent toward each other to form a closed loop. Consider the story of Anna as portrayed by Dr. Abigail Zuger in her April 14, 2014 *New York Times* essay, "Too Much Family Love." As a well person, Anna would go for her routine checkups alone at the end of a day at work. But then Anna became seriously ill. As Zuger writes,

> *It turns out she had one of the great families of all time, a big cheerfully intertwined conglomeration... From the moment she was hospitalized they never left her side. Or, more precisely, they never left her by herself...there is actually a bit of a difference between the two.*

The problem is not just that Anna can't ever be alone, but she must make the most critical decisions about her care among family members who refuse to allow her to give up. Rather than disappoint them, she chooses to go along with their wishes, prolonging but not bettering her life.

It's hard to define the right dose of family. It shifts from day-to-day, as does the specific concoction of family we want and what we need them for. And while we are in the midst of illness and caregiving we are needed by others, another child, an aging parent, a disturbed spouse. We come to illness with habits and history that affect the medical experience and are worthy of exploration.

Writing Prompt

- Pick out the family members who are critical to your story. Before incorporating them into your narrative of illness, create profiles of them by showing them in various scenes and situations. This is as much to help you understand them and your relationships as it is to provide background. Put yourself into the scenes to show the interplay between you and them. What are the strengths and weaknesses in your relationship? What baggage do you carry? Write about your shared history, past moments of transformation or alteration.

- Write specifically about your family of origin. If it helps, describe your childhood home, where you slept and ate and went to read a book, the sound of slamming doors when you fought (my sister's door always made a satisfying slam while mine was more like a Volkswagen, some act of air pressure never allowing the door to close completely), what you heard in the middle of the night. Show you and your family going in and out of these various rooms, the shifting of attentions and tensions, joys and grief.

• Now write about the role of family during illness, whether you were the one being treated or the caregiver. Who defined those roles? How did illness affect your relationships? Use dialogue, anecdotes, large and small family interactions, scenes between family members and doctors. Write about issues of privacy and intrusion, the wresting or giving of control, distance or avoidance, regression into old roles and patterns versus new ways of relating.

• Create a family tree based on actual lineage. Now draw a new one where the closeness or distance between relations is based upon the importance of that person to you, i.e., an aunt who is more like a mother should be closer, a sibling with whom you are feuding should be on an outer limb. A best friend may be on the same line as a brother or sister.

• Were there times when you were denied access to a family member because, for example, a hospital didn't recognize the rights of a same-sex partner, a feud kept someone you loved from visiting, children were not allowed, ICU rules limited who could visit and when?

The Third Thing

I married John right out of college. It wasn't because I was ready to be married. More accurately, I wasn't ready *not* to be married. I met John the first week of my freshman year. We had two months to get to know each other before I was assaulted by anxieties and drawn into a depression that extended through our entire four years at school. John cared for me, incorporated my phobias into our plans, brought me home to his mother. He drove us from New York to Pittsburgh to see my sister because I was too afraid to fly and gave me math problems to solve to distract me from the dizziness and tremors I felt in the no-man's-land between departure and destination. When we married he drove me to my flute lessons, did the grocery shopping, took me on elevators and subways to get me used to them. John took care of me and catered to me for four more years before I found my own strength.

Building a new dynamic required the construction of new scaffolds, modified floor plans, different finishings. But this took time. We worked in different worlds, we had different tastes in music and movies, different friends, different ideas of where we wanted to live, different religious and cultural backgrounds. At times I felt as if we parallel played through the earlier years of our marriage.

"Third things are essential to marriages, objects or practices or habits or arts or institutions or games or human beings provide a site of joint rapture and contentment." This quote by Donald Hall from his memoir *The Best Day the Worst Day* never ceases to strike me with its obvious brilliance. For many years it seemed as if my husband and I didn't have a third thing. Children, of course, became our third thing, but raising our children underscored our divergent roles and perspectives. But third things pushed themselves up through the loam of our marriage. John came to the opera with me and learned to love it; I was as eager to travel to Ireland to visit his relatives as he was. We loved the sea—he to sit by it, me to immerse myself in the salt water; we went to the mountains to ski. After years of walking in Central Park by myself or with a friend, John started coming with me. For a couple of years, *Hardball with Chris Matthews* was a third thing, so was Charlie Rose. Now it's kabbalah class and learning how to row.

Illness is a third thing, although no more welcome than a nighttime intruder that makes a couple cling to each other. If the intruder stays too long, though, the third thing can split and take on a different form for each member of the couple. There might be a difference of opinion on the best way to deal with the intruder. One of you may want to beat it, the other to learn to live with it. One may want to call for help, the other to handle things on his or her own. The third thing may be seen as a bigger threat for one of you.

Illness can be a third thing one day and not the next.

Writing Prompt

- If you are part of a couple, write about the third things that have arisen for you during your time together. Show you and your partner engaged in those shared pleasures that existed before illness and how those third things have changed and evolved over time. Was it a struggle to find those third things or did they always just seem to be there? Were there times when there seemed to be no third thing?

Now, write about illness entering your life whether you are the caregiver or the person afflicted or, perhaps, both. What parts of yourself have been activated—your bitterness, compassion, spirituality, sense of humor, need to control, etc.? How has your partner reacted? What common ground do you share and where has the ground shifted beneath you?

- If illness was always present in your time together, explore in what ways it brought you closer and in what ways it pulled you apart. What are the third things you share that have nothing to do with medicine or doctors or disability or illness?

Cast of Characters

The doctor said..., the nurse swabbed..., the technician arranged..., the orderly entered..., the receptionist looked up... Who are these people—the doctor, the nurse, the technician, the orderly, the receptionist, the social worker, the security guard, the anesthesiologist, the ambulette driver, the physical therapist, etc.? These people are in your story. They may not all be crucial to the plot but, like the extras or small roles in a movie, they are the context in which the action takes place. I was once given a piece of advice about character writing; even if you will never show that person having breakfast you should know what he or she would eat. Even if a sibling may never make an appearance in your story, you should know whether your character has one. Why does it matter? It matters because how we ultimately write about a person depends on how well we know him or her—idiosyncrasies, appetites, hometown, relationships, favorite attire, sleeping habits. Our characters, fictional or not, become real by discerning what all these details are.

Nadia had two primary doctors. Since they filled different needs in both me and Nadia it was important to distinguish them, not just visually but by their characters. I never learned what either one had for breakfast, but I did learn about their families, religious beliefs or lack thereof, pets, experiences they had when they were young, the kind of jokes they liked to tell, what events in the world mattered to them, etc. I didn't know as much about less-significant characters, but when I wrote about one of Nadia's nurses I knew about an upcoming wedding, where she was from, the similarity in her background to that of my husband and his sisters. All these details made me feel tenderness as I wrote. In the case of a hard-edged nurse, I was struck by how she never smiled, even with her colleagues. I imagined her eating toast and grapefruit for breakfast, the citrus leaving her lips pinched all morning.

Writing Prompt

- Make a list of everyone you came or come into contact with on a routine basis. Next to each name write everything you know about that person, whether or not you think he or she is central to your story. If there is a person about whom you know little but realize more information would make your narrative deeper, think about how you can fill in these blanks. For the major characters, create a profile for each one including appearance, the sound of their voice, favorite phrases, gestures or tics, the smell of soap, sweat, aftershave, or alcohol swabs. Include what you might know about the person's family, religious beliefs, favorite foods, pets, former careers, professional training, favorite books, etc. You will not write all of this information in your story, particularly details that aren't yours to share, but they will put meat on the bones of your characters.

It isn't just patients who want to be treated as individuals. Those on the medical/service side do as well. Notice any changes in your attitudes toward the people you interact with once you start wondering about their breakfast choices.

What Friends Are For

Nadia was diagnosed and, in an instantaneous work of alchemy, I was no longer the same as my friends. The facts of Nadia's illness littered the path between us like bear traps. They would tell me I was so strong; I would tell them they would do the same. They all gathered at the hospital the day of Nadia's surgery; I took strength from their presence but was too focused on using my psychic energy to keep Nadia alive to talk to them. They were sure to ask me every day how I was; I didn't want to look too closely at how I was doing and Nadia still had cancer. What else was there to say? While I didn't know if I wanted them to bring food, flowers, or just their familiar faces, I did know I wanted to be seen by them as the person they have always known.

When my father was diagnosed with Alzheimer's disease, the only alchemy was one which bonded me even more tightly to my friends. Being in a social group with other fifty-five- to sixty-five-year-olds meant I had an automatic support group. They all knew my father and came the day of his funeral. We talked and told stories and ate good food.

"You need your friends not just as friends but as corroborators," Julian Barnes observes in his book *Levels of Life*. Barnes' wife had died and he worried that his memories of her were being altered by time and emotion. This worked for me during my father's illness but could not during Nadia's.

The role of friends in times of crisis is one of those black holes of etiquette. In a beautiful meditation, *A Grief Observed*, the author C.S. Lewis writes about companionship on the opening page. "There is a sort of invisible blanket between the world and me. I find it hard to take in what anyone says. Or perhaps, hard to want to take it in. It is so uninteresting. Yet I want others to be about me. I dread the moments when the house is empty. If only they would talk to one another and not to me."

Writing Prompt

• Write a variety of scenes that include you and your friends. Think of the times when your friends were most valuable and of when the relationship floundered. Write about how your friends responded when you told them your situation, when you were in the hospital, when you had to cancel a lunch date, etc. Pick one or two friends and write about how your relationship with them has evolved.

• Did you make new friends within the world of illness—perhaps someone in a support group, a waiting area, or with whom you shared a room? Has the friendship lasted or do you think it will?

• If you had to write a guide for friends of people undergoing a medical crisis of their own or of a loved-one, what would you say?

They Said What?

Eat a healthy diet, exercise, do puzzles, get outside a lot and you won't get Alzheimer's disease. *My father was a marathon runner, an outdoorsman, an inventor with a genius IQ who wrote his own puzzles to solve; for years before he died he couldn't tell time, figure out how to open a milk carton, or speak a sense-making sentence.*

You're so strong. I couldn't do what you're doing. *Strong is when you choose to accept a burden, not when you have to.*

Don't worry; you'll still look good in a sweater. *My mother's lips formed a tight line; she had told her neighbor about her mastectomy and this was the woman's only response.*

Wow. Look at that cute little body. I wish I was so slim. *You could be if you went through seven rounds of chemotherapy and had your jaw rebuilt and couldn't eat solid food for six months.*

When you tell people you are ill, are getting divorced, have lost a job, are having a baby, have experienced a death, you are going to hear a lot of advice and "wisdom." It will range from silly to harmful to hurtful. Everyone will hear from a person with an aunt or cousin who went through the same thing, who has an alternative treatment to recommend, who has some religious perspective to share.

The words come from family, friends, colleagues, strangers, and even medical professionals. In *Autobiography of a Face*, as Lucy Grealy faces the prospect of surgery after surgery to reconstruct her disfigured face, her doctor tries to sympathize by saying everyone is unhappy with some part of how they look. "Why, he himself had terrible acne as a teenager," he shared with Grealy, "and that made him feel awful. Acne, was he serious?"

The need to say or do something in the face of a fellow human being's strife is admirable, but no one wants to be made the property of another person's ideas and imaginings.

Writing Prompt

• Write a poem or list of all the inappropriate or hurtful comments people have made in response to your illness or that of someone you are caring for. What did you say or wish you had said? Suggested opening lines might be: Don't tell me..., I don't want to know..., He said, she said, they said..., People say..., My sister's friend said..., It's time..., You should..., You'll see... Below, as an example, is Rose Garland's poem, *Personal Questions*, inspired by Diane Burns' "Sure, You Can Ask Me a Personal Question." It appeared in the Fall 2013 of *The Healing Muse*, a literary and visual arts journal of the Center for Bioethics and Humanities at SUNY Upstate Medical Center. This is the format the author chose; you can create your own or, if you want, adapt this one.

> *No, I'm not a smoker. No, I never have been.*
> *Yes, it's one that smokers get.*
> *No, I'm not a heavy drinker. No, I never have been.*
> *Yes, it's one that drinkers get.*
> *Yes, you can say it's unfair.*
> *No, I don't see it that way.*

No, this isn't a punk haircut.
No, this isn't a perm.
No, it wasn't curly before.
No, I don't want to wear a wig.
Yes, I could get one on the NHS. A pretty one. A
good one.
No, I don't want to wear a scarf.
Yes, I could get one on the NHS. A pretty one. A
good one.

No, I haven't tried multivitamins.
Or selenium.
Or coenzyme Q10.
Or folic acid.
Or beta-carotene.
Or coffee enemas.
Or broccoli.
Or linseed.
Or the Gershon technique.

Ah, so you have an aunt with cancer.
Ah, your brother.
Yes, it's the same as Michael Douglas.
Yes, things have moved on since you were a boy.
Yes, there's a better chance these days.
Yes, it's amazing what they can do.

Thanks for saying I look well.
No, I don't feel it.
No, I don't like it when you squeeze my hand.
Or hug me.
Or stroke my hair.
And say it's soft as a baby's.

Yes, these electric wheelchairs are useful.
Ah, so you think they're brilliant.
Ah, so you'd like one yourself to get about.
No, I don't think I'm brave.
Really, I don't see myself as brave.
No, really.
If you must, then.

No, there's nothing you can do for me.
No, there's nothing you can do.

- What were the most helpful responses from both friends and strangers?

- Were you ever the one dispensing advice to others? What were some of the comments you made which you wish you could take back?

Sense and Sensuality

College, for me, was a time of deadened and distorted senses. The ground never felt solid under my feet; standing still felt like balancing atop a raft in a rough ocean. Food had turned gray; my body refused its entrance. My eyes no longer thirsted for nature; despite the full moons and the changing foliage of the seasons outside my dorm, my eyes stared instead at my walls of cement blocks. I thought I could no longer sense beauty. But I still had music, the only medium which moved me beyond my body when the rest of the world was drained of its color.

The sound of the voice in song was the only sensory experience in which my mother found transformation in her final year, when she could no longer eat the salty and vinegary foods she loved, when a swim in the ocean could only be imagined, when her hands could no longer immerse themselves in the dirt of a garden. As writer, philosopher, and cancer survivor Mark Nepo says in his book, *The Exquisite Risk*, "… song is not a luxury but a necessary way of being in the world, of keeping the soul anchored in hard time, a way for each of us to experience the fullness of life, no matter what difficulties we wake in."

Eating is another experience of the senses. It was one of the few left to my father who could no longer read, understand or make speech, or enjoy running his hand across a piece of wood he had just sanded. Dining might have become difficult for him but he still responded to flavor and texture. He also responded to visual beauty. On a summer visit to his home in the mountains of New Hampshire a year before he died, my father called me over as soon as I got out of the car to look at his orange rhododendron bush. It was a striking plant, startling in the sunshine against the backdrop of distant mountains. Our mutual enjoyment of the sight was a moment of communication between my father and me.

Writing Prompt

• Hearing, sight, touch, taste, smell. Write about moments when your senses were engaged or were lost. Which senses did you value most before illness; which ones offer you the most transcendence now?

• Write about a specific meal. If it was at home, write about the preparation, setting the table, the dishes used, who was there, what was on the menu. Relay the conversation or the silence. Who cleaned up? Maybe the meal was interrupted before everyone was finished. If the meal was at a restaurant, give details of the setting, what you ordered, what you wore, who you were with, the occasion, your comfort level, how you felt on the ride or walk home.

• Lovemaking is a primary and primal sensual experience. Write about the impact illness has had on physical intimacy and drive.

- Write about a time before illness when music or another art form transported you, brought you from one state of mind to another. Show yourself turning to music, theater, dance, literature, or art after a day at work when you were ready to give notice, had a fight with a friend, slogged through rush-hour traffic. Write about the physical sensations within your body. Do the same during a time of illness, caregiving, or grief.

- Set aside twenty to thirty minutes to immerse yourself in your art form of choice. For example, if it is music, close your eyes and, without analyzing, allow yourself to feel how your body and heart are responding. Let your thoughts float by without comment. When the music is over, take five to ten minutes and, without pausing or lifting your pencil from the paper (or fingers from the keyboard) write whatever comes to mind about the experience.

I Know

A mother who participates in the Children's Museum of Manhattan's Shelter Program for Families in Temporary Housing where I teach wakes in the middle of the night and feels the loss of not knowing the stories of those who came before her. "How many women and children have been here before?" she asks. "I wonder what the walls would say? How much laughter have they heard? How many tears have they seen fall to the ground?" She wants to know these women.

Even in small moments of discomfort we want to hear, "I know." If I wake up in the morning dizzy, with my sinuses aching, I tell my husband and if he says, "I know, I have to turn my head so slowly when that happens to me," I relax. The adage goes, "Misery loves company." But a bunch of people sitting around saying how miserable they are is not the same as saying, "I know." I know how you feel as you sit in the waiting room. I know what it feels like to have your mind muddled by morphine. I know what it's like to use the handicap-accessible lift on the bus for the first time with all those people staring at you.

There's a reward, too, for the person who says, "I know." When we offer our voice to another, we create compassion within ourselves. Compassion, I have found, provides a coating for our overwrought nervous systems. It eases pain's grip—our own and that of others.

Writing Prompt

•   Imagine that you are writing to a person who you can understand intimately, not because you know him or her but because of common experience. Pick a moment—waiting for a diagnosis, a first treatment, a conversation with a family member, being in a hospital or other foreign place, a moment of isolation or boredom—and begin to write. Think of this as writing little vignettes or making a small painting. Imagine the person to whom you are writing finding your note on a chair in the waiting room, inside an MRI machine, on his or her bed at home, etc. Make your writing visual, show actions and gestures that reveal what is occurring, include internal dialogue, bring in noises and sights from the world outside the window or door of the person to whom you are writing. Here is a brief example of what I would say to a mother in a waiting room:

I know you don't really want to talk right now, particularly to a stranger. Talking requires control of your breath and I know you can't really do that beyond the little sips you are taking, enough to keep you from blacking out, although what a relief that would be—to forget for a moment what is happening. That's why I left this note on your chair when you got up to get a magazine. There's nothing in that dated TIME that will hold your interest, but it's good to have something to hold and busy your hands with. If you're like me, you're afraid that if you take your focus off your child, you won't be able to save her. I see you jump each time a name is called or a doctor or nurse enters. Don't worry, you will hear them over the sound of CNN. What war are they talking about now? What pop star has made a fool of himself? What weather disaster has struck? We all get sucked into the TV, even at times like this. You are not neglecting your child. She's probably playing with the latest app on your phone anyway. Your day here will be over soon. Then the sun, which you can see only out the sliver of window, can warm your shivering bones. Then you can take your daughter and run.

- Here are some ways you can begin: I know you are…, I can see you…, I have been where you are…, If you're like me…, I have been there…

- Write what you wish you knew, what you don't or didn't know, what people around you did or didn't know.

- Write about a time when you felt no one knew you, when you felt as if you lacked definition because there was no one to see you at your moments of greatest vulnerability. Try writing in the third person, or as if you were directing a scene for a movie—moving from a close-up, where it is just you, and then slowly panning out to include other characters, the room, the world outside. As a filmmaker, you must think about mood, lighting, dialogue, sound, action, etc. How do your feelings alter as more of the world enters? To whom would you like to say, "Know me now, in this moment"?

Retreats and Rituals of Comfort

I grew up in a house that abutted conservation land and my favorite place to hide was in the woods, out of view of my house, underneath the branches of a beech tree. I didn't go there just to cry or pout. If that's all I wanted to do, I could have gone to my room, closed the door and shed my tears into my pillow surrounded by my menagerie of stuffed animals. Rather, I was looking for a way to soothe myself, and the need to be in nature was primal. I inhaled the scent of the earth; I ran the dirt through my fingers. I listened to the wind and felt it brush my neck. I followed the growth of the leaves as they went from bud, to green foliage, to autumn hued, to a blanket on the forest floor. Nature became a lifelong source of comfort that I thought would never fail me.

What soothed us in the past may not provide the same comfort now. When Nadia was ill, nature had lost its healing touch. It was the man-made world that was healing Nadia and I began to view nature for the impersonal force that it is. It is twelve years later and I am still figuring out the role of nature as a source of comfort. I know I still crave its beauty and force; my Martha's Vineyard home still captivates me with its views of ocean, pond, bird- and sea-life. But solitude no longer nourishes me; I am searching for a new balance between the comfort of people and the embrace of nature.

Writing Prompt

• Was there a place you went to as a child, a ritual you enacted, or an activity you engaged in that soothed and comforted you? Describe your retreat. What kind of events sent you in search of solace?

• Have your sources of comfort changed over time? Write about the healing place or practices you turn to now. Are you still searching for what can soothe you?

• Retreating into places of comfort can exclude others. Have you ever used these places as a means of keeping someone outside of your life? Have you ever felt excluded by someone who has retreated into his or her pain?

Sacred Time and Spaces

I do not believe in God. I wish I did. It sounds like it would be so soothing, like playing that game where you fall backwards knowing that your friends will always catch you. But through my religion, Judaism, I am constantly seeking to add depth, meaning, and compassion to my life. I have fallen into pockets of what I can call sacred. It happened one Friday night when Nadia was in the hospital. My older daughter had joined us. We lit the Shabbat candelabra (no real candles allowed). We ate our dinner by its glow. We spoke in soft murmurs. Nadia fell asleep. I thought I could hear the far-off rustle of the Sabbath Queen's robes. But I flinched. Visitors came, the lights were turned on, the next episode of "Survivor" appeared on the TV. The Sabbath Queen was voted off the island.

She returned, briefly, several months later at Frannie's bat mitzvah. It was held outside by the sea on Martha's Vineyard. The ritual was an acknowledgment not only of Frannie's maturity, but of the place we had come to as a family following Nadia's illness. So what made the day sacred, what made me fall in love with the *Mi Sheberach*, which calls for the healing of body and soul, came not from a core belief but from an already heightened emotional state that, like a dye, seeped into the fabric of our observance. I would love to have faith, but what I seek now are sacred moments in whatever form they come.

I think this is why I loved Mark Doty's beautiful narrative on the death of his lover from AIDS, *Heaven's Coast*. He begins with a rumination on religion. "I don't know what I want in a church, finally; I think the truth is that I don't want a church."

Doty isn't saying he doesn't believe in awe or the sacred. "Wind, glimmering watery horizon and sun, the watchful seals and shimmied flurries of snow seem to me to have far more to do with the life of my spirit. And there is somehow in the grand scale of dune and marsh and sea room for all of human longing, placed firmly in context by the larger world: Small, our flames are, though to us raging, essential."

The themes of religion, faith, what is sacred, the magnificence of the natural world are ones that the memoirist of life-altering experiences always confronts. They arise in the question of why, in the search for sources of strength and compassion, and in the quest for respite from disease. We wonder about religion when people say, "God only gives you what you can handle," when we receive Mass cards, or someone calls to say they said a *Mi Sheberach* (a prayer for healing) in synagogue. We know what isn't sacred—either the ways in which our churches, temples, and mosques fail us or the ways our secular culture does. Maybe rituals that once held so much meaning before we were hit by a crisis show themselves to be no more real than a hologram. But crisis can also transform so that the plaintive call to prayer of the muezzin, for example, becomes a call to open one's heart.

Writing Prompt

- What is your relationship with religion? Write the scenes from childhood that marked your early experiences with ritualized observance and faith. What role has religion played throughout your life? Describe the places that felt sacred to you and those that didn't. Write about the ways, if any, your religion or faith has become integrated into your experience with illness. Are there rituals or religious guidelines that you have turned to or away from? Have you ever bargained with God?

- Write a healing prayer, or other kind of prayer.

- Play architect and design a sacred space.

Animal Therapy

After I heard the words, "Nadia has cancer," after I asked what kind and will she live, before I knew what would come to matter and what wouldn't, I thought about my dogs. Would they be a threat to Nadia's compromised immune system?

"Can we keep them?" I asked.

The doctor said they could stay; they could even be therapeutic. I knew he was talking about how they could help Nadia, but it was me I was worried about. The dogs my family had at the time were mine, adopted when my children were babies. One was just a puppy when I was pregnant with Nadia and her twin brother Max. The shelf made by my bulging belly was her favorite place to perch. After I gave birth, she found a new perch on my shoulders as I nursed my babies, and one in my heart. She became my shadow and partner. She watched me eight years later as I cared for Nadia, as if reassuring me that what I was doing was right.

Over twenty years later, it was through three other dogs that I was able to communicate with my father as his dementia progressed. Never a fan of pets of any sort and never what I would call gleeful, he would turn giddy with joy watching my dogs run. He insisted they come with us everywhere, and they gave him security on our walks in the woods; he trusted them more than me to find the way home.

I wasn't surprised to read in Mark Doty's memoir *Heaven's Coast* that he brought home a new puppy months before his lover, Wally, died. "[Wally] could barely use his hands then…but he's reaching over with his barely functional hand to stroke Beau's neck."

In *Autobiography of a Face*, the author Lucy Grealy describes a similar relationship with horses.

> *The horses remained my one real source of relief. When I was in their presence, nothing else mattered. Animals were both the lives I took care of and the lives who took care of me. Horses neither disapproved nor approved of what I looked like. All that counted was how I treated them, how my actions weighted themselves in the world. I loved to stand next to them with no other humans in sight and rest my head against their flanks, trace the whorls in their hide with the fingers of one hand while the other hand rested on the soft skin of their bellies. All the while, I'd listen to the patient sounds of their stomachs and*

*smell the sweet air from their lungs as attentively
as if I were being sent information from another
world.*

For many, it is through an animal that we first experience the cycle of life, from conception to birth to aging to death; animals help us practice our ability to be nurturing and compassionate. In our animals and how we treat them, we can see a reflection of ourselves.

Writing Prompt

• Tell your animal stories. What is/was the role of animals in your life? In what ways, if any, are/were they a source of comfort, distraction, or normalcy in the face of illness?

• If you didn't or don't have a pet of your own, write about any animal encounters you have had. You can write about trips to the zoo, a safari, snorkeling over a coral reef, birdwatching, or your experience growing up or working on a farm.

• Have you had any experiences with a pet therapy animal? If so, write about that experience and what it meant to you. Do you think animal therapy is a valuable supplement to medical care?

Greedy Hearts

My father had Alzheimer's disease. There's nothing good I want to say about that. He was a genius who graduated with a Master's degree from MIT when he was twenty-three, who no longer knew what a number was, who built his own boat but no longer recognized the word for what he created, who taught me about nature and the sky and ended up thinking clouds were just crazy, who was a marathon runner who had to be held and coached to walk or sit down. My father left us bits at a time and remained aware enough to recognize each time a new piece flaked off.

I am not a person who believes there is a purpose behind everything. My father didn't get Alzheimer's to teach me about himself or myself or my family. I can't spin this into gold for the soul. And yet...

The elevator door opens and I see my father sitting in a chair in the hallway opposite the nurses' station waiting to be taken for a haircut. I greet his physical presence but must work a great deal harder to find his mental one. When I do, his response to me is pure love, the kind of unconditional joy in my arrival that I used to get from my children when they were little and now get from my dogs. It has been this way since those brain cells I used to imagine crammed into my father's skull began dying and leaving others to drift. Not that I didn't know already that my father loved me. But he held his love loosely enough so I would be free to live my own life.

Now, my father is holding onto this love more tightly so I relish this hello, as well as the goodbye when he shows me he knows he is still my father in ways he never did before—more touch, more tears. His heart has opened not just to his family but even to my dogs and to any child who crosses his path. A former marine, he wants only peace and can't even look at a picture of a gun. To this father, I press my forehead against his after kissing him goodbye. He says, "Be careful. Take care of yourself. Do you have money?" New words from an old father. I want to remember this man as much as the one who loved me in his sanity.

In her novel, *Tell The Wolves I'm Home*, Carol Rifka Brunt writes in the voice of a fourteen-year-old girl who has lost her uncle to AIDS and is about to lose his lover whom she has only recently gotten to know, as well:

> *And then I thought something terrible. I thought that if Finn were still alive, Toby and I wouldn't be friends at all. If Finn hadn't caught AIDS, I*

would never even have met Toby. That strange and awful thought swirled around in my buzzy head. Then something else occurred to me. What if it was AIDS that made Finn settle down? What if, even before he knew he had it, AIDS was making him slower, pulling him back to his family, making him choose to be my godfather. It was possible that without AIDS I would never have gotten to know Finn or Toby. There would be a big hole filled with nothing in place of all those hours and days I'd spent with them. If I could time-travel, could I be selfless enough to stop Finn from getting AIDS? Even if it meant I would never have him as my friend? I didn't know. I had no idea how greedy my heart really was.

Our hearts are greedy—greedy for anything positive we can take away from a horrible situation.

Writing Prompt

- Write about what, if anything, your greedy heart filled itself with during a time of illness or trauma. Show a time of joy or breakthrough or deeper communion that occurred through the experience of being a patient or caregiver. Some might find gratitude in these moments, others bitterness. What do you feel?

What Now

"After mothering with such intensity, what do I do now?" Nadia had had her final chemo; all that was left was to get through the side effects, the scans that would confirm she was in remission, and then the removal of her central IV line. As I stood outside the procedure room in the hospital for this final operation, I had daymares that the horrible thing I had been waiting all these months to happen was finally occurring. Perhaps the doctors were trying to resuscitate my daughter from some one-in-a-million disaster as I waited. I did not know how to stop myself from being an exaggerated mother. Nadia awoke from the anesthesia with no physical harm done, but she too seemed at a loss to define who she was now. Reluctant to leave the hospital, she stayed in the playroom for a while doing the activities she had become so familiar with.

My question of what to do now was premature. "The past six months cannot be stowed away, removed to the attic with other artifacts of history." But Nadia's hair would grow back, she would return to school. Her illness had become a room I had lived and worked in with no distraction; now I was being told I could open the door, but my feet resisted stepping over the threshold. The landscape outside was filled with gaping holes of empty time that I might fall into. I couldn't imagine how I would fill them up.

Writing Prompt

- Write about time suddenly opening up for you. It could be at the beginning of health and survival, it could be after a death, it could mean a caregiver has had to place a loved-one in a long-term care facility and no longer manages the daily needs of the patient, in the case of a chronic illness it could mean an acute phase has been resolved or additional help has been obtained and the time spent devoted to the illness is much less now. Compare your fantasy of what you would do once you had time with what the reality is like.

- Examine the relationship between you and a caregiver/the person you were caring for. Are you moving forward in synchronicity? Write about old patterns versus the new ones you may or may not have established yet. Describe the first time you were alone without the person with whom you shared the experience.

- Think of metaphors for this sudden freedom to use time as you wish, i.e., time is a house with no walls, a fifth season, a bungee cord that promises freedom and then snaps it away.

- Go back in the past to other moments when time opened up for you. Think of when you graduated from school, summer vacation, when you retired, when your children were gone from home. What is similar between these moments and the time when you became free from the daily demands of illness?

The Phantom Road

I never thought very much about the title of the well-known Robert Frost poem that begins, "Two roads diverged in a yellow wood," and ends with the lines, "I took the one less traveled by, / And that has made all the difference." It could have been Two Roads or All The Difference. All I thought, at the time, was that it was a poem about choice and what mattered most was the road that was taken. The other road seemed to no longer exist. But the name of the poem is "The Road Not Taken." So is Frost telling us that the path we don't travel is as significant as the one we do? I began lingering on the third stanza which includes these lines: "Oh, I kept the first for another day! / Yet knowing how way leads on to way, / I doubted if I should ever come back." The paths we don't travel, particularly when we are diverted from those paths by events outside of our control, are ghosts that haunt us, taunting us with thoughts of what might have been if we had turned left, right, or backward; if illness hadn't barricaded our way.

We can't say for sure that the person we become by traveling one road would be the same or different if we had taken another. It seems useless to ponder. And yet I do. I can assume that having cancer has somehow helped shape Nadia into the person she is today. But how can I parse the ways in which her essential self has been sculpted by illness versus all the other events and influences in her life? Before age eight, Nadia was defined by her confident strut. I was always behind her, following her lead. She kept that strut during treatment, but afterward she began to wobble. Entering adolescence, she lost so much momentum she almost toppled, but what teenager doesn't struggle anyway? Was every weakness and vulnerability I saw in her a side effect of cancer?

I analyzed everything. Would she have remained a gymnast and never found her passion for dance? Would she have had different friends, acted up a little more? Would she have gone to a different college? Nadia's spirit wants to see the world, but her adventurousness has been restricted by anxiety. Where might she be now if she could set herself free? What would our bond be like, since it was during her treatment for cancer that I finally began to understand my little girl? I could create many narratives of what might have been. But that seems unfair to Nadia. She is who she has become and I love every inch of that person. Drawing a portrait of some other girl named Nadia would be a betrayal.

It is easier to imagine how my path would have been different. I softened during Nadia's illness, dropped a good deal of my moralizing. I laugh more now. On the old path I imagine there would be more fights around the dinner table as I lectured on my latest goals for my children's behavior. On the old path, I would feel sorry for myself whenever the kids or my husband joined together to tease me or argue against me. It made me feel separate from them. I don't allow that to happen anymore. I either talk back or shrug it off. I don't cling to my children anymore or need their existence to define me, a good thing since they are all now in their twenties. The biggest question for me, though, is where I would be as a writer; perhaps I would have found my way to the literature of illness through some other experience, or maybe I would be writing fiction or wondering why write at all?

Writing Prompt

• We can never know exactly what would have happened on the road not taken, but we can imagine it anyway. Write a scene or scenes from your life as if illness had never struck. Think about the ways in which you used to interact with others, your mannerisms, your tone of voice, the things that got you riled up, what made you laugh. Think about the objects and ambitions you had; picture yourself in the job you hoped for, the direction of your marriage or other family relationships. Your scene can be around a dinner table, in the car, on the subway, shopping, at school, on a trip, etc.

• As you write, note the ways in which you see yourself as changed or influenced by your or a loved-one's illness. Which changes do you welcome; which do you regret? Can you see where the two different roads merge and diverge?

Part III

Inside the System

Medical practice is a many-tentacled being—each arm a system of its own. Your doctor's office has a system, your hospital, American health care in general. You become tangled in insurance systems, communications systems, systems for keeping records, delivering medications, deciding on protocols. Technology is a fast-growing tentacle; small-town, community-based practice in many cases an atrophied one. This is your chance to write about what it is like to be wrapped in those tentacles, whether they feel like a comforting hug or a straightjacket.

Systems are man-made contrivances. They create a layer, often opaque, between you and the experience you are having or the person you are relating to. Like illness, systems can take control away from us. But unlike illness, they have their roots in human actions and decisions and so we respond differently. We have a chance to change them, no matter how remote and how little energy we might have for actually doing so.

In this section you will still be writing from your personal experience; indeed, many of the scenes and feelings you uncovered in earlier chapters will inform much of what you write here. But now you have the opportunity to examine how you function within a system. What makes sense to you? What makes you want to slam down the phone or rip up your paperwork? Are you a rebel or a conformist? You can write about what you did or wish you had done when the tentacles overwhelmed you. You are encouraged to offer opinions on what worked for you and what didn't. You can suggest solutions and make suggestions, use skills you might have (or didn't know you had) in planning and design. You may end up writing an op-ed piece or, if you find an issue of particular interest, you may find yourself writing in a more journalistic vein, what is often called creative nonfiction, using your own experience and those of others to report on a state of affairs you believe needs more attention.

Be creative in how you approach these chapters. Some will call for straight narrative but others will allow you to play architect, designer, or policy maker. All, I hope, will help you realize the power you have not only to convey the experience of illness but to influence how care is provided and received.

The Good Doctor

Every year I help to judge an essay contest for medical school students sponsored by The Arnold P. Gold Foundation for Humanism-in-Medicine. The prompts vary from year to year but the crux of each one is to show or define the good doctor. Enormous attention is paid to examples of compassion—eye contact, taking time with the patient, listening to the patient's story. Some essays focus on small gestures—adjusting the sock of a patient under anesthesia, a reassuring touch, providing a bottle for an undernourished, crying baby. Others depict doctors who travel to underserved communities where their selfless gestures impact the most destitute. In essence, the essays speak to healing rather than curing. No one writes about educational credentials, hospital placements, research projects, academic posts, or honors and awards.

Dr. Danielle Ofri, an associate professor at New York University School of Medicine and editor of the *Bellevue Literary Review,* writes about her own experiences practicing medicine. In an October 5, 2013, opinion piece in *The New York Times,* Dr. Ofri writes about a patient whose glucose levels were dangerously high. Together, they came up with a plan for lowering them. The patient would eat one fruit or one vegetable every day. "A perfect example of shared decision making," Ofri writes.

But then Ofri checks her past notes and discovers the same agreement had been made on each prior visit. "Each time," Ofri says, "I must have congratulated myself on the excellent patient-centered care." So is the good doctor the one who follows the rules of humanism-in-medicine, or the one who, like Ofri, evaluates her success or failure?

Nadia had good doctors but, beyond their exemplary credentials, they had little else in common. One doctor conveyed so much kindness I almost didn't care if he had a medical degree; another doctor made Nadia laugh and feel like her opinions about the world mattered. One surgeon made me feel as if we were teammates— not a doctor and a patient's mother; another surgeon made none of those soothing small gestures but wasn't above developing respect for Nadia's spirit. They saved Nadia's life. But that's not what made them good. It's that they so deeply *wanted* to save her life.

Writing Prompt

• What is your definition of "the good doctor?" Support your definition by showing examples of the good doctoring you have experienced or witnessed. By detailing specific scenes with the doctor, illustrate the qualities that are important to you. Show the small gestures that do or don't matter. Write the conversations that you had, not just the words but the tone of voice, the eye contact, the inclusiveness. On rounds, did the doctor use your name with his or her cadre of trainees? Did you care? Did you know the doctor's credentials?

• Do the same exercise with the disappointing or bad doctor.

• Write about a favorite nurse, therapist, volunteer, child life specialist, or anyone else in the medical community who has impressed you.

• Write a letter of recommendation for your "good doctor."

• Pretend you are the doctor's supervisor and write up an annual review.

The Good Patient

I used to say doctors were responsible for the quality of the doctor/patient relationship. The patient, after all, is in need, vulnerable, wrapped in confusion and fear. Why add another layer of concern? But even in sickness we can still find those pockets of self from which we can give. In Anne Fadiman's *The Spirit Catches You and You Fall Down*, the doctors who treated the dire illness of the daughter of a Hmong immigrant family never received one word of gratitude, never felt as if the family reached as far as they did to bridge the divide between them. In this case, the cause was an extreme cultural dissonance. Even as I know and understand this, I couldn't help but feel compassion for the doctors. Their desire to heal emanated from an internal source, but it was only natural for them to want some external acknowledgement of how hard they were striving on behalf of the family's little girl.

The fact is, many of us want to be good patients, but how we define that term is not the partner to the definition we give of the good doctor. From the good doctor we have expectations; the good patient is a plea. Here is what Mark Nepo writes in *Surviving Has Made Me Crazy*: "I'm almost polite, accepting ill treatment in order to be seen as good and kind. I feel, all too often, that if I say the needle has been put in badly, I'm causing trouble or being ungrateful or complaining. Worse, there have been times I've pretended there isn't even a needle in me, so as not to hurt the one poking."

I was recently engaged in a conversation about whether the labels of doctor and patient demean the patient, implying an imbalance of power. I've heard people advocate for the terms provider and patient, or client and consumer. Time Warner is my cable provider; I am my lawyer's client; when I call the plumber I receive a service; I am a customer at my local bookstore. None of these exchanges come close to reflecting the relationship between a doctor and a patient, even when it isn't at its ideal. The physician has hard-earned knowledge that I don't have. While I believe patients and families must be informed about health care, part of my end of the partnership with the doctor, once I have put myself under his or her care, is to commit to that person; to ask questions of course, but to be compliant when a treatment plan is prescribed. (Too bad compliant sounds so much like complacent.) And I want to be kind, to ask about the family photo on the desk or say "thank you" when a doctor or nurse takes extra time with me. Even my father, five days before his death from Alzheimer's and barely able to speak or interpret his surroundings, used his moments of clarity to thank the woman who washed his hair, to say hello to a nurse entering the room.

Writing Prompt

- Write a definition of a good patient. Think about the Hippocratic Oath. Create a similar oath for patients.

- Write about a time you were not a good patient. This does not mean a time when you were legitimately angry because of bad treatment or callousness, but when you didn't hold up your end of the doctor/patient relationship. What were the circumstances? What would you have done differently?

- Write a thank you note to a favorite medical professional. Send it.

Healing Hands

The hands that are supposed to heal you are often clicking on a mouse or scrolling down a screen, looking into your body on a laptop while you sit on the examination table, or maybe they're not even in the room at all. Palpation, the method whereby a doctor uses his or her hands to form a picture of the internal state of a person's body, is also a time of human connection. Touch is so powerful we would shrivel without it. Yet here the doctor's hands palpate a computer. The technician who took the pictures had to hide behind a shield or exit the room leaving no hands within reach. During her diagnostic process, Nadia spent the entire day at MSKCC getting scans. At some point, maybe after the MRI and before the bone scan, we came upon her surgeon, an actual person, in the hallway. For a few minutes, he was an oasis.

Nadia's scans were necessary. Palpation could not determine the extent of Nadia's cancer, or, by the time it could have, it would have been too late. But the need for a scan isn't always so obvious. There was disagreement among Nadia's own doctors about what scans she needed three and five years after treatment.

Too much data can be confusing. Mammography saves some lives and creates unnecessary panic in others. A blood test that shows an elevated PSA can send a man into a similar tailspin. You can go to the Mayo Clinic and get your entire body scanned and have your blood analyzed for conditions you barely knew existed. What do you do when a spot shows up, when "out of the range of normal" appears on your printout? Is it significant, or would it have just sat that way forever, you happier being none the wiser?

Science is an unstoppable system. Humans will always ask questions and look for their answers. In the abstract (and as a scientist's daughter), I find that very exciting. But genome mapping, 3-D imaging, the generation of actual flesh, all raise practical and ethical questions we have barely begun to address. What would seem obvious to some, that a cochlear implant would be a blessing for a hearing-impaired person, engenders the opposite reaction in others.

Writing Prompt

- Write about the various ways doctors have looked inside your body. What did it feel like to be on the MRI table or to be stuck with a needle and looked after by technicians whom you never met? Did you think all the scans and tests you had were necessary? What happened when you expressed concern or refused a scan? In what ways, if any, did testing affect your relationship with your doctor?

- Write about a time you were confronted with having to make a decision based upon test results which were ambiguous?

- If you have an opinion on tests like mammography, that look into the bodies of usually healthy and low-risk people to identify a problem, write an op-ed piece based upon what you have experienced.

Bits and Bytes

In the practice of medicine today, the doctor and patient are joined by a third party—technology. Robotics has entered the operating room; electronic medical records and computerized checklists streamline information keeping and sharing, knowledge (and often incorrect knowledge) is within reach of anyone with a computer. When Nadia began her treatment, the examination rooms at MSKCC's day hospital were so small that personal connections were unavoidable. There were no computers in the rooms. Communication was through eyes and ears. In the present day, computers are ubiquitous and it is up to the medical professional how that computer will be used. These machines do not contain narrative but sets of data. For all of their benefits, there is a concern that doctors depend on them too much, believing a snapshot needs no accompanying story.

I'm curious about how technology has affected the doctor/patient relationship and the practice of medicine. At a lecture at Wesleyan University, Dr. Rita Charon, the physician who founded the Narrative Medicine program at Columbia University, presented a portrait of the computer as a physical barrier to personal and visual communication between a doctor and patient. Buttons needed to be pushed and fields entered—a patient's words translated into code. The Arnold P. Gold Foundation for Humanism-in-Medicine reported on a small study indicating that patients stop their narratives while doctors are interacting with their computers and continue only when there were gaps in computer usage.

It isn't just computers in the medical setting that impact our relationship with a doctor. How many of us have been able to resist the lure of WebMD or the bottomless well of medical information, or misinformation, that can be found online? It is now possible for us to have made our own diagnosis and treatment plan before we even register with the receptionist at the doctor's office. It's likely we have Googled the doctor. And, in his January 16, 2014, article in *The New York Times*, Dr. Haider Javed Warraich tells us our doctor may have Googled us, as well.

Now, along comes IBM Watson™. Maybe you know it as the computer that beat two of Jeopardy's greatest champions. But Watson, which is programmed to use and respond to language like a person, is poised to perform serious work in the medical world. Its job is to take the patient information and test results gleaned by the doctor, match it up with a store of information on up-to-date research and treatment options no doctor could keep up with or store in his or her own brain, and arrive at a ranking of possible diagnoses. It's easy for me to see the value in Watson, of having access to so much information, just as, taken individually, we can see the value in robotics, medical imaging, electronic medical records. But we still need a relationship between the doctor and the patient who are already swimming upstream through bits and bytes to connect to each other, to reveal not just the medical story but the human one.

Writing Prompt

- Write about your experiences with computers and technology. Was there a time when a computer created a barrier between you and a doctor? In what ways do you value technology; what ways has it seemed unnecessary or impersonal? If your doctor(s) used a computer while you were telling your story, write about what that felt like for you. Describe the doctor's office, where the computer was placed in relation to where you and the doctor were sitting. Include what kind of eye contact you had, the sound of the keyboard, any other devices (cell phones, beepers) that might have interfered with your conversation.

•   I didn't search the Internet about Ewing's sarcoma until after Nadia finished treatment. It was not a search for helpful information or to make me a wiser consumer. It was to prove that what we did was right, to hear over and over what her odds were, to confirm yet again the credentials of her doctors, and to stay connected to a year of living so intensely. How have you used the Internet during the course of your illness or caregiving? Show yourself at the computer, your sweaty and shaky fingers, what is coming up on your screen? Share interactions you might have had with others in the same situation. When you finished your session, what were the physical sensations in your body? Did you feel reassured or more anxious? Did it affect your trust in your doctor? How often, if at all, were you drawn to the Internet?

•   How would you feel if you found out a doctor Googled you? Can you think of an occasion when it might be beneficial?

The Fourth Amendment

Privacy is so valued in our society that our highest court interpreted the Fourth Amendment of the Constitution to mean that it is our right. Since 1996, a patient's right to privacy has been protected by The Health Insurance Portability and Accountability Act. This includes the HIPAA Privacy Rule, the Security Rule, the Breach of Notification Rule, and the Patient Safety Rule, all overseen by the Office of Civil Rights.

But what does privacy mean when our bodies are exposed to doctors, nurses, technicians, people in hallways who pass us as we lay in beds waiting for "transport"? What is privacy when curtained enclosures around beds restrict sight but not sound or smell? What is privacy when your body shows on the outside the effect of your illness or condition and everyone feels they have as much right to study you as they would a piece of art in a museum? What is privacy when we can claim no HIPAA protection against the questions of family and friends? What is the impact of all this intrusion?

In *Truth & Beauty: A Friendship*, about her relationship with the late author Lucy Grealy, Ann Patchett writes, "Every scar was a badge of honor, and she was always pleased to whip off her shirt to show someone the scars on her back and tell their unhappy story. She had a lack of physical modesty common to many people who had spent that much time naked in hospitals."

Nadia is the opposite; she has always guarded her privacy and still does. Ask her too many questions or point a camera at her for too long and the shield she will erect is almost visible. It rebuffed the doctors who invaded her privacy and provoked her pain. But her shield was porous; like a sunshade, it hid the part of herself she wanted kept secret but it could not prevent the intrusion to her eyes and ears. I became her blackout shade. Too often, I forgot this part of my job. After her diagnosis, Nadia began to get a lot of cards. When she opened the first one she cried, "You told people?" I started to tell her I had to, but I couldn't help her understand why. I had to give what was happening to her and our family a voice, but to Nadia I had undermined one aspect of her life she could control: who should be told and when.

There were also times I failed to protect Nadia because I was too busy gawking and eavesdropping on this unfamiliar world I was suddenly thrust into with the absorption of a tourist in an exotic land. In *Motherhood Exaggerated*, I write:

Nadia is halfway through her day of chemo when I pick up the middle of a conversation between the girl in the bed next to Nadia and her social worker. The girl is perhaps nineteen. I come in on these words: "You know, you're out of treatment options."

"Yes, I know," the girl answers.

"Have you thought about what you want to do in the time you have left?"

"Well, I want to keep going to school for as long as I can."

"Good, you should feel better for a while since you won't be getting any chemo.

"I'm looking forward to hanging out with my friends."

"What about when you can't go to school anymore? Do you know who's going to take care of you? Are you talking to your doctor about palliative care?"

I am fascinated by this conversation, with the girl's calm acceptance, with the fact that she has no mother or father there to make the conversation easier. Or maybe her parents would have made it worse. How could they not project their despair?

But I also don't want to hear anymore. I don't want Nadia to hear it. I turn the television volume a little louder, ask Nadia if she needs anything or wants to play cards. I fuss with the items on the bedside table. I try to make noise to block out the voice of the girl who is going to die.

Writing Prompt

- Write about moments when you felt your privacy was invaded. Choose scenes from both before and after illness. Has your need for privacy changed? Have you become more or less willing to reveal hidden aspects of yourself? Include details in your scene that convey the emotion of the moment.

- Write about the moments when you had glimpses into the private lives of others. If you write about a stranger, show in your scene how it felt to gain such an intimate view of someone you didn't know. If it's a family member or a close friend, show how trespassing on their privacy, either accidentally or purposefully, made you feel.

- Write your own HIPAA regulations.

- Every writer, particularly of memoir, must wrestle with the ethics of sharing the intimacies of another person's life while telling his or her own story. While honest and open exploration benefits readers, the writer has a great responsibility to respect his or her characters and to get their permission before making any writing public. The writer must also be certain that any information that is included must be necessary to the story being told. Be aware of this potential paradox as you write about privacy.

Medicine as a Second Language

How far into your brain can the words penetrate when the doctor says, "Your child has cancer," "All your symptoms point to MS," "You have diabetes and we have to start you on a treatment plan right away"? The words have no trouble finding their mark in your heart and soul but your brain has only been grazed. It's why we are advised to bring a less-involved person to those doctor's appointments when a diagnosis is delivered, a treatment described, or a surgery recommended.

Nadia's doctor told us not to take notes during our early meetings. He wanted our attention on him. He promised he would repeat himself many times, which he did. Slowly, my husband and I learned what we would need to know, or what we thought we did until my sister-in-law would tell us what we hadn't heard.

In the growing field of Narrative Medicine, doctors are taught the art of taking a history so that they can write the patient's story in all its facets, not just the outward specifics of what has brought the patient in that day. But the doctor has his or her own story to tell, as well. Narrating the diagnosis, the treatment, the side effects, the time frame, the impact on home and family—this is the tale a doctor must tell. But often there is no way to measure what is heard. After hearing the details of Nadia's treatment, chemotherapy every three weeks, I still thought she would be able to go to school in-between infusions, even after I heard the doctor talk about fevers and low white-blood-cell counts and mounting exhaustion.

In one of the leading works on the potential gap that can exist between doctor and patient, *The Spirit Catches You and You Fall Down*, author Anne Fadiman deconstructs an extreme case of cultural clashing through the story of Hmong refugee Lia Lee and her parents, and that of the Western doctors trying to treat her epilepsy. As one of Lia's doctors noted: "It felt as if there was this layer of Saran wrap or something between us, and they were on one side of it and we were on the other side of it." I knew how fortunate we were that Nadia was treated at a leading hospital in our home city, that we spoke the same language as the doctors, and that we had a preexisting understanding of the medical system and hospital procedures. Others—because of a language barrier and despite the hospital's interpreters, or because of cultural conflicts or mistrust, or perhaps because of an inability to comprehend a series of complex tasks—would, in the language of doctors, be labeled noncompliant. Mothers in the outpatient area changed the dressing over the implantation site of their children's central IV line. We had been warned not to perform this task in the hospital with its multiplying germs. Some mothers did not create a sterile field, or they would eat their lunch while swabbing the site. I didn't understand this. The task was stressful, but the instructions were clear. But sometimes we just don't hear, or understand, or remember, or are not told why it matters. We are given so many chores to perform, unlike any we ever had to complete before, it's impossible to keep track sometimes.

Writing Prompt

- Write a scene or scenes when you felt swamped by information or unable to understand what you were being told. What kind of impact did this have on your ability to care for yourself or to be a caregiver? Was it hard to ask the doctor to clarify a point? Did you feel as if you were imposing on him or her? Was the doctor available? What role did the nursing staff play in helping you to absorb information? Was there a social worker or a patient advocate you could turn to? Write your suggestions for improving the communications process.

- Did you experience any cultural or religious collisions or times when your traditions or rituals were in contradiction with what the doctor wanted you to do? Did you have access to interpreters? Were you able to find others within your culture from whom you could learn? Which, if any, of your beliefs or lore, were challenged or altered?

- Since even the best doctors can't see everything, we can use our stories to assist them as healers, to challenge assumptions, to recognize that the experience you are having is layered and opaque. Think about moments that arose or have arisen during treatment for an illness or disability or while being a caregiver. What would you want a doctor, nurse, or other medical professional to have seen?

Define Dignity

"The quest to achieve true dignity fails when our bodies fail." This is a quote from the late Dr. Sherwin B. Nuland's book, *How We Die*. He wrote the book because he felt conversations about a "good death" and "death with dignity" didn't take into account the realities of what he saw. His aim was not to scare readers but to prepare the ill or their loved-ones so as not to be alarmed or guilty when faced with a death in which a failing body does not simply drift away. As Gary Shteyngart describes his Grandma Polya's death in *Little Failure:* "She is dying in parts, as most of us do. Skeins of hard-won adulthood peeling off."

Hospice has become the holy grail of the "good death," either at home or at a hospice house. I had never experienced this form of palliative, non-interventionist care until my father was admitted to hospice when his Alzheimer's disease reached its end stage. He entered disoriented and agitated. But visitors would come and say at least he was at peace now. Peace? In his bed my father bicycled his legs, flailed his arms, tried to rise, talked to himself or invisible others, and made expressions that ranged from a smile to pain to terror. Dignity? We discussed funeral plans over his bed, having been told he couldn't understand us, as if he were the forgotten child who hears all the fights and secrets in the family.

What people meant was that the setting was peaceful. The hospice workers cared for my father with the mindfulness of Zen Buddhist monks. Even when they knew he was going to die within an hour or maybe two they bathed him and trimmed his mustache and put soothing balm on his dry lips. They were like external dignity pumps.

I am grateful for hospice. It gave my father the best possible death. But it is a mask for the violence that occurs at life's end. When the mask came off I found my grieving complicated. I could not say that what happened was good. Rather than wrestling with tangled notions of dignity, it is more accurate to say that what we are seeking at the end of life, or at any stage of illness, is compassion.

Writing Prompt

• Write about your experiences with dying—whether you were at a loved-one's bedside or a distance away. How did what happened support or contradict preconceived notions on how you hoped that person would die? Set the scene. Where were you? Who else was there? What sounds did you hear? What did people say? Was it calm or hectic? Could you describe it as a good death?

• Respond to Dr. Nuland's belief that we lose dignity when our bodies fail.

• What expectations, fears, anxieties arise for you when you think about your own death? What is your belief about what happens when you die?

• Have you written a living will? If not, write one now. Don't just include advance directives regarding lifesaving measures, write about who you would want to be present, where you would want to be. My mother planned her funeral—the speakers, the music, where her ashes were to be buried. If you want to, and think it would be helpful to you or your family, write down a guide for your own funeral. If you need help having these difficult conversations, I recommend visiting www.theconversationproject.org.

Tell Me Where It Hurts

"How's the pain today?" This is the first question my physical therapist asks me about my neck and jaw pain. "What number would you give it, on a scale of one to ten?"

"Ah, a six?" I might answer. I don't really know what a six is. I think a ten would be so excruciating that I wouldn't even be able to make it out of the house and a one would be no pain, not even a twinge. *Five*, I say to myself, *would be my average and I'm a little worse this day, so a six*. But a five may not be someone else's average, so it feels meaningless.

"The insurance company might not reimburse for a six," my PT says.

"Okay, a seven then." I don't really feel like I'm cheating because if I don't get therapy the pain would become a seven or even and eight, so I'd still need treatment.

Children are often asked to look at faces to describe their pain, from smiling to neutral to frowning to crying. "Can you tell me which face looks like how you're feeling?" the doctor or nurse asks. Maybe the child will pick a face with a downturned mouth but no tears because he or she is in some pain, but not enough to cry; or maybe the child picks the frown because he or she is still unhappy about a sibling who "borrowed without asking" a brand new toy.

What about the question, "Where does it hurt?" I could answer, "It hurts in my jaw," but the hurt in my jaw might be from a hurt in my heart or a nerve in my shoulder or maybe I need a root canal. Ask any parent with a child who complains of a tummy ache and you'll hear how hard it is to pinpoint the precise place of pain.

So, while pain management has earned greater attention as a necessary part of medical treatment, pain itself remains a relative quality. It fluctuates. It may be fickle in its response to treatment. It is as much about perception as it is about fact.

Writing Prompt

• Create a system that doctors could use for assessing pain. It could be an extension or modification of existing methods or it could be a brand new one. Think back to the chapter on metaphor to see how this literary device might be used.

• Write about your experience trying to describe your pain to others or about trying to decipher someone else's pain. What words or gestures were used? Write about the feeling of being in pain or of watching a loved-one who is hurting. Was/is your pain managed well? What worked or is working for you? What do you think is still missing in the management of pain?

• How accessible were alternative methods, i.e. acupuncture, meditation, yoga, biofeedback, homeopathy? If you used any of these methods, did you find them helpful? How do you think the traditional medical establishment could better incorporate alternative strategies into traditional treatment?

The Ideal Hospital Room

Lucy Grealy was in the fourth grade when she entered Ward 10 at what was then named Babies Hospital in New York City to begin treatment for a Ewing's sarcoma. In her book, *Autobiography of a Face,* Grealy describes the ward—its green and gray tones, the worn patches on the floor, the wooden doors, the bars on the windows. "I was always a fan of the gleaming new," Grealy says, "but in time I came to find this dinginess comforting, more humane than the fascinating but alien landscapes of newer wards I would later visit."

Since the early seventies, when Grealy was a patient on Ward 10, hospital design has entered a new era. Nadia was part of that transition at the MSKCC. In the seven months of her treatment, the Pediatric Day Hospital went from a communal ward of curtained-off beds to a temporary facility with separate, semiprivate rooms, to the current facility, opened in 2001 just after Nadia finished treatment, which offers private rooms and so much natural light the staff complained about the heat and the glare. On the inpatient floor, where once only those with severely compromised immune systems had the "honor" of being isolated, all of the rooms are now private.

Nadia and I had differing views on the merits of having a roommate. I wanted only solitude, to not hear the muffled weeping of another mother or the unmuted cries of her child. Nadia was looking for a friend, another traveler on the road she was on, someone to go to the playroom with, someone who could give her a feeling of a social life. I think Grealy would have been in Nadia's camp since she seemed to thrive on the company and comradeship of the other children on her ward.

So I thought of Grealy and Nadia when I came across an article announcing the design of Patient Room 2020. With support from the Department of Defense, NXT Health created a room meant to alter the medical experience to reflect the knowledge, technologies, and innovations of the twenty-first century. It is sleek and hi-tech, hinting that its designer has spent more time than most of us in an Apple store. You can view the room at nxthealth.org/portfolio/patient-room-2020/. Visit the site before you go to the prompt.

Writing Prompt

• What did you think of Patient Room 2020?
Now you be the designer/architect of what you would
consider to be the ideal hospital room. Don't let
your creativity be limited to size, furnishings, color
scheme, lighting, and aesthetics. Think about sound
and noise, storage, interface with other patients, and
with the medical staff. Consider minimizing the risk
of infection and falls, of increasing a patient's sense of
independence. Redesign the bed if you see a need there.
How would you incorporate technology? A patient who
is mobile may want someplace to sit, eat, read, or watch
TV other than the bed. What would you design? What
about a place for a family member to sleep? Would a
man need a different kind of space than a woman, a

child than an adult? When Nadia was in the hospital I brought her blanket from home, her favorite stuffed animals, pictures to decorate the walls. What would you do to make a room feel like home? Do you think that's important? Should a hospital room be a place where medical procedures can/should be performed?

• Clip inspiring pictures from magazines, draw a floor plan or a blueprint, create a model.

• Design other spaces. Perhaps your home needs adapting because of a medical need or maybe you have a new perspective now that requires a new aesthetic. Redesign your bedroom or kitchen or create a room you've never had before. How about a writing room!

Insurance

I bet that one word, insurance, is enough of a prompt to get you writing. Maybe you have a positive story to tell or maybe you are just waiting for a chance to rant; in either case, insurance goes with illness the way report cards go with school. We were fortunate during Nadia's treatment. Fending off an insurance company nurse who wanted to share with me her wisdom on how to treat Ewing's sarcoma in the event the doctors at Memorial Sloan-Kettering didn't know what they were doing was a small price to pay for Nadia's excellent coverage. It was confusing, though, that after her treatment the insurance company insisted they knew of no person named Nadia Hannan whenever I tried to file a bill. Maybe they thought they had done their share.

There is no doubt that the trail to reimbursement can be circuitous and rocky, with blind curves and dead ends, and with the futile hope that the music played while holding for "the next available representative" would change to a song you liked. Choosing among the options of how we are covered and by whom, what doctors we can see and how much we pay, is only getting more complicated. Even as we must become literate in medicine, we must spend our draining emotional and intellectual reserves on research, calculations, and paperwork.

Writing Prompt

•   Write an opinion piece on the insurance climate based upon your experience—both good and bad. How would you improve it? In what ways was treatment affected by your coverage? Were there times when a less expensive option existed (i.e., at-home care versus hospitalization) for which you could not get reimbursement?

•   Write a phone conversation you had with an insurance agent.

•   If you didn't/don't have insurance, write about how that impacted treatment and your financial well-being. Have you tried to get insurance but couldn't? What kind of insurance system would you like to see?

Appendices

Quick Prompts

Here is a list of phrases or suggestions for you to respond to. Don't overthink these. Respond to the first thought that arises. You can do any of these multiple times.

What matters

I used to be… but now I'm…

In the heart of me you will find

If you should meet me upon the street

I have a question to ask you

Write a monologue of some part of your body (i.e., if your leg could talk)

Have you forgotten me?

That was the time when

What if/if only

Write about your name

Write a letter to your older self; write one to yourself as a child

If it weren't for

Write about a time you felt powerful

Write your earliest memory in the child's voice; no

reflection or fancy words. Now write it from the age you are now.

If you loved me you'd

The people I used to know

Write about a moment during the past week you don't want to forget

What I should have said was

Write about what you are wearing

The best day of the week

The first time

I am from

This is how it is/This is what happened

Good enough

When time stood still

I thought I knew you

Write a telephone conversation

Make a list of possible opening lines for your story

Take a sentence from a favorite book and use it as your opening line.

Behind closed doors.

You/He/She/They never told me

An Ending and a Beginning:
Where Are You Now?

At the beginning of this book, you set out on the journey of your own story. Perhaps you followed the chapters serially; perhaps you skipped around; perhaps there are chapters that you haven't explored. However you got to this point, here you are. Where is that? Remember the second chapter on "Getting Here"? How would you write that now? What have you found on the path you just traveled? What are you still looking for? Are you comfortable at this place to which you have arrived?

Now is also a good time to think about why you write and whether or not your motivation and purpose has changed at all. Whether you began as a novice or a practiced writer, you have honored your voice and therefore yourself. For whose ears is that voice intended? It could be you have written only for yourself, to find understanding, meaning, and/or transformation in what you have gone or are going through. You may also have written as a way to share with family and friends, for no matter how close these people may be to us, we still must guide them to see beyond the surface of our daily lives. Finally, you may be seeking a wider audience for your writing—to help others who have experienced what you have or to reach the wider range of committed readers with the universality of your story.

Your travels, of course, have not ended; *The Write Prescription* can be your companion as your story continues to unfold. Repeating exercises, choosing different prompts, and writing from chapters you passed over the first time around will all help you go more deeply into your own thoughts and mine more material. Each time you arrive at a new place, your perspective changes. You have matured, examined old grievances in new ways, connected with friends and loved-ones on different terms. I urge you to continue to challenge yourself to tell your story.

I wrote *The Write Prescription* as a resource for moving through and beyond the experience of illness by creating narratives around what has occurred. It is not a guide to writing for publication. However, rereading and revising your work can be a way of opening up more of your story. If you are interested in refining your writing for any reason—for your own self or because you are interested in publishing—your will find a few tips in the following pages.

After the First Draft

My first drafts are often more like skeletons than full-bodied pieces. It is during the revision process that I add muscle, tissue, hair, and clothes. But I do not approach this challenge in a linear fashion. I might carve a right bicep and then be drawn to the left foot, which needs a sock. While fattening up the gut I might already be thinking about adding a pair of pants. But before buttoning them I'll get distracted by time and decide to add a watch. Applying eyeliner and lip gloss, I'll feel something nagging at my thoughts until I look and see I never finished the right foot. And when I finally think I'm finished—I've buttoned the pants, chosen a shirt, tucked it in, and strapped on a belt—I'll realize I've forgotten to put on underwear.

The point is, our first drafts are just that. Drafty. They can be full of holes, or they can be full of thoughts and information blown in on the winds of memory that, while valuable to you, may clog up the piece you want to write. First drafts may not close properly. They can get stuck. It sounds like a contradiction, but this can be particularly so if, in your initial writing, you do what you're supposed to do and uncouple your gut from your brain and let the words flow without judgment or censorship. But if you want to create a more polished piece, it's time to apply a more evaluative eye and ear.

In what follows you will find some tips for rewriting and refining your work. While creating publish-worthy pieces is not the specific intent of *The Write Prescription,* reviewing your work can help you unearth new thoughts and ideas, to go more deeply into your subject, to dress your skeleton. So use as many of these tips as you wish, either solely for the purpose of mining your topic more fully or also to make the writing itself stronger. These tips are not exhaustive; they are not meant to take the place of a writing class or workshop, but they can work as an adjunct to more participatory settings.

Time is Distance

You've written your first draft, maybe read it through once for obvious errors. Now, put it away. Work on another piece, practice the piano or your French, take a road trip—engage your mind with other topics and activities. After a week or two, take your piece out and read it with a fresh eye. What remained hidden before—the non-sequiturs, the gaps, the dropped storylines, the repetition of words and phrases, etc., will now be more obvious.

What's It About?

Now that you have read your piece, can you say what it is about? You must be able to answer this question if you want to proceed any further. A story isn't about what happened, it's about the impact of events and how you or others were transformed. If you haven't arrived at this transformational moment, you still have more writing and delving to do. If you can answer the question, your editing and revisions must support that point.

Read Aloud

When we use just our eyes to read we can miss a great deal. We bunch words and phrases together, skim whole sentences, rush the rhythm of the words. When we read aloud, we give weight to every syllable. We discover a cadence and can feel when it becomes disturbed. We stumble when words don't fit together smoothly or a sentence has an awkward construction. Sometimes, we find ourselves drifting into a monotone because our voices have been lulled by sentences that are all the same length and construction. Notice the spots where you stumble and phrasing is ambiguous. Think about word choice. Which works better—couch, sofa, or divan; syringe or needle; empty, vacant, or vacuous. A word isn't just its definition; it is its sound as well. Reading aloud also is a different emotional process than writing. Notice where your eyes tear and your throat constricts, or when you remain unmoved or confused.

Tighten, Tighten, Tighten

Be ruthless in your editing to make sure that every word has a purpose and supports what your work is about. In our insecurity, we often say the same thing multiple times in different ways to make sure we have made our point. Trust yourself that you have made your point and trust your reader to understand it. Notice digressions. Sometimes we can be so fascinating to ourselves when we're not necessarily to others. A beautifully crafted sentence, full of richness and metaphor, that has nothing to do with what you are writing about, has no luster. Delete it.

Use Action Words

Which sounds better? 1) When the doctor came into the room she saw I was in pain and decided to increase my pain medication; or 2) The doctor entered and gave me a shot of morphine. I hope you chose number two, particularly if, in the sentences before, you created a vivid scene of the pain you were in. The first choice stops the action while the second one maintains the momentum. It's not unusual to write in a more passive voice when facing traumatic experiences. It protects us from the pain. But in a second draft, where you have already achieved some distance, it is easier to spot and change these moments.

Show Don't Tell

This old saw again. In the chapter called "This Is How It's Done," one suggested prompt was to show yourself doing something like brushing your teeth or fixing a drink when you are angry or sad or excited. This is what is meant by showing rather than telling. Look for moments when you say something like, "I was so angry when I went to bed," and write more deeply into what that was like. "My hands were shaking when I tried to put the top back on the toothpaste. I gave up, throwing the tube, the top, and my toothbrush into the sink. That felt good. I grabbed my slippers and pitched them overhand into the closet, slammed the door, whipped back the duvet on the bed (the ugly one from my ex-mother-in-law with the pink roses on it), and mashed my head down onto the pillow. Ugh. Maybe I'll dream about revenge."

Be Specific

Are you including details in your writing? Check to see that you have enough of a physical description of your characters that they can be imagined. When you write about a meal, include what was eaten, its aroma, its texture; write any conversation that was had. Details are what will bring your scene alive. If a room is painted blue is it navy, sky, or royal? Go back to the chapter on "The Five Senses" and see if you are using what you learned there.

Time Is Distance (Part II)

Put your piece away, again. Wait as many days as it takes until you're not thinking about it anymore. Then read it again, silently and aloud. Go through the checklist of tips. Refine again.

Other Readers

This suggestion should be accompanied by a big, red caution sign. You have done all that you can on your own and would now welcome another set of eyes and ears. But your writing is a piece of you, a naked you, and the wrong reader can send you back under the covers. You are looking for feedback, not criticism. You want the person who will say "I loved it when you said...," and "I was a little confused about...," and "I'd love to know more about the time when..." Make this very clear to the person you hand your writing to. Your first reader probably shouldn't be your spouse, or your mother, or someone who has a different view of events than you do. It may not even be your best friend. Be open to what you hear. It's natural to be defensive. I know I am. But if you let that feeling go, and the comments you receive are constructive and supportive, your writing will only get better. If you are thinking about joining a writing group or class, apply the same philosophy of feedback, not criticism.

I would love feedback on your experience with *The Write Prescription*. Please contact me through my website, judithhannanwrites.com. Thank you for sharing this journey with me. I wish you luck as you continue.

Bibliography

Bailey, Elisabeth Tova. *The Sound of a Wild Snail Eating.* Chapel Hill: Algonquin Books, 2010.

Barnes, Julian. *Levels of Life.* New York: Vintage, 2014.

Broyard, Anatole. *Intoxicated by My Illness.* New York: Fawcett, 1993.

Brunt, Carol Rifka. *Tell the Wolves I'm Home.* New York: Dial Press, 2012.

Cahalan, Susannah. *Brain on Fire.* New York: Simon & Schuster, 2013.

Doty, Mark. *Heaven's Coast.* New York: Harper Perennial, 1997.

Fadiman, Anne. *The Spirit Catches You and You Fall Down.* New York: Farrar, Straus and Giroux, 2012.

Grealy, Lucy. *Autobiography of a Face.* New York: Harper Perennial, 2003.

Hall, Donald. *The Best Day the Worst Day.* New York: Mariner, 2006.

Junger, Sebastian. *The Perfect Storm*. New York: W. W. Norton and Company, 2009.

Kushner, Rabbi Harold S. *When Bad Things Happen to Good People*. New York: Anchor, 2004.

Lewis, C. S. *A Grief Observed*. New York: HarperOne, 2015.

Lopate, Phillip. *Portrait Inside My Head*. New York: Simon & Schuster, 2014.

McCourt, Frank. *Angela's Ashes*. New York: Scribner, 1999.

Mukherjee, Siddhartha. *The Emperor of all Maladies*. New York: Scribner, 2011.

Nepo, Mark. *Surviving Has Made Me Crazy*. Fort Lee: CavanKerry, 2007.

Nepo, Mark. *The Exquisite Risk*. New York: Harmony, 2006.

Nuland, Dr. Sherwin B. *How We Die*. New York: Vintage, 1995.

O'Brien, Time. *The Things They Carried*. New York: Mariner, 2009.

Patchett, Ann. *Truth & Beauty: A Friendship*. New York: Harper Perennial, 2005.

Price, Reynolds. *A Whole New Life*. New York: Scribner, 2003.

Rapp, Emily. *The Still Point of the Turning World*. New York: Penguin, 2014.

Shteyngart, Gary. Little Failure. New York: Random House, 2014.

Theroux, Paul. The Tao of Travel. New York: Mariner, 2012.

Acknowledgments

Bouquets of gratitude to Nancy Aronie—my first teacher, my always teacher, my forever friend; Catherine Barnet—who makes me believe I am talented enough to be her colleague in teaching and writing; and Nancy Kelton—the first person to introduce me to the idea of the "aha" moment.

Thank you also to the friends and associates who have encouraged me in the creation of this and other work: Patty and Doug Sacks, Patty Newburger and Brad Wechsler, Dr. Maureen Strafford and Alex McDonald, Cathy and Salvatore Trentalancia, Jackie Clason, Elizabeth Doon, Leslie Bushara, Dr. Michelle Friedman, Dr. Ramon J. C. Murphy, Dr. Angela Diaz, Rabbi David Ingber, Andrew Ackerman, Judith Kelman.

Joan Cusack Handler, Publisher and Senior Editor of CavanKerry Press, who, in the process of making *Motherhood Exaggerated* the best book possible, raised my writing to a new level. She continues to be my cheerleader.

To my communities—the Mount Sinai Adolescent Health Center, the Children's Museum of Manhattan, the Arnhold Global Health Institute at Mount Sinai Icahn School of Medicine, Congregation Romemu—who have showed me how to love and live more fully.

To every student I have ever had, it is an honor each time to hear the words of your heart.

Lisa Weinert and Tyson Cornell are the founders of Archer Lit and a dream team for any writer. I am proud to be part of your exciting venture. And to Kate Sage, thank you for your insightful editing skills.

I owe thanks to my sister and brother-in-law, Dr. David and Joan Roth, for so many reasons. To keep things simple I'll just say I'm grateful for your bottomless and unconditional love.

John, Frannie, Max, and Nadia, you are the ultimate for me. I am grateful every minute for the light with which you imbue my life. It never dims or dulls, nor does my love for you.

Judith Hannan is the author of *Motherhood Exaggerated* (CavanKerry Press, 2012), her memoir of discovery and transformation during her daughter's cancer treatment and her transition into survival. Her essays have appeared in such publications as *Woman's Day, The Forward, Opera News, The Huffington Post, The Healing Muse, ZYZZYVA, Twins Magazine,* and *The Martha's Vineyard Gazette.* She teaches writing about personal experience to homeless mothers and at-risk adolescents as well as to medical students, and is a writing mentor with the Visible Ink program which serves patients at the Memorial Sloan-Kettering Cancer Center. She is a judge of the annual essay contest sponsored by the Arnold P. Gold Foundation for Humanism-in-Medicine. She served as Director of Development of the 92nd Street Y and then for the Children's Museum of Manhattan. She now serves on the board of the Museum and on three boards affiliated with the Mt. Sinai Medical Center in New York—the Adolescent Health Center (where she now serves as President of the Advisory Board), the Children's Center Foundation, and the Arnhold Global Health Institute. She lives in New York.